When Altruism Isn't Enough

The Case for Compensating Kidney Donors

Edited by Sally Satel, MD

The AEI Press

Publisher for the American Enterprise Institute

WASHINGTON, D.C.

Distributed to the Trade by National Book Network, 15200 NBN Way, Blue Ridge Summit, PA 17214. To order call toll free 1-800-462-6420 or 1-717-794-3800. For all other inquiries please contact the AEI Press, 1150 Seventeenth Street, N.W., Washington, D.C. 20036 or call 1-800-862-5801.

Library of Congress Cataloging-in-Publication Data

When altruism isn't enough : the case for compensating kidney donors /
    edited by Sally Satel.
        p. ; cm.
    Includes bibliographical references.
    ISBN-13: 978-0-8447-4266-3
    ISBN-10: 0-8447-4266-X
    1. Kidneys—Transplantation—Economic aspects. I. Satel, Sally L.
    [DNLM: 1. Kidney Transplantation—economics. 2. Kidney Transplantation—
    ethics. 3. Tissue Donors—ethics. WJ 368 W567 2008]

    RD575.W54 2008
    617.4'610592—dc22

                                                            2008045715

12 11 10 09 08   1 2 3 4 5

Printed in the United States of America

To Virginia and Steve Postrel

Contents

List of Illustrations

Acknowledgments

As with all books, particularly those with multiple authors, many people have contributed their time and ideas to this publication; we are grateful to all of them. The contributors to this volume have put countless hours into wrestling with these complex questions, and have benefited from the advice of many other fine scholars.

In early 2007, Sally Satel of the American Enterprise Institute approached Richard Epstein of the University of Chicago Law School about the feasibility of holding a conference at the University of Chicago, cosponsored by their respective institutions, to explore the many questions related to compensating organ donors. At that conference, which was held in July 2007, the contributors to this volume presented early drafts of the papers that are contained within this volume. They received valuable comments and criticism both from their fellow authors and from others in Chicago who were active in the issues surrounding organ transplantation.

The contributors to *When Altruism Isn't Enough* wish to acknowledge all those who helped with the book in numerous ways. The success of the original conference at the University of Chicago stemmed in large part from the organizational skills of Marjorie Holme, the coordinator of the law and economics program, and the editing of the papers produced by it was undertaken by Sally Satel, Samuel Thernstrom, and Lisa Ferraro Parmelee at the American Enterprise Institute.

For editorial assistance, the authors wish to thank Tal Manor, Mary Knatterud, and Stephanie Daily. For research assistance we are most grateful to Jonathan Stricks and superb AEI interns Adam Hepworth, Emily Sands, and Michelle Sikes. Others who provided invaluable research support and editorial assistance were Grisel Gruiz, Christopher Levenick, Samuel Gregg,

Kyle Vander Mulen, Paul Eggers, Joel Newman, Guiliano Testa, and Paul Kimmel. Richard Epstein wishes to thank David Strandness, Stanford Law School, Class of 2007, Paul Laskow, New York University, Class of 2009, and Michael Schachter, New York University Law School, Class of 2008 for their excellent research assistance. The chapters also benefited greatly from critical reading by Mark Cherry, J. Michael Millis, Michael Novak, Robert Sade, and James Warren, and discussion with Joseph Antos, Robert Helms, and Alex Pollock.

For generous institutional support, deep thanks go to Dean Saul Levmore at the University of Chicago Law School, Dean Deborah Powell at the University of Minnesota Medical School, and Dean Guy Charles at the University of Minnesota Law School. The National Institute of Aging provided a Career Development Award (K23-AG021963) to Elbert S. Huang, which was greatly appreciated. Sally Satel gratefully acknowledges the support of Howard Palefsky, Victoria Palefsky, and Rose Marshall for this project.

Introduction

Sally Satel

In June of 2007, a Dutch TV station announced an upcoming real-life program featuring Lisa, a thirty-seven-year-old woman with an inoperable brain tumor. During the show, Lisa would select which one of three needy contestant-patients would receive one of her kidneys after she died. Though only Lisa would pick the lucky winner, viewers could express their preference by voting over the Internet.

News of *The Big Donor Show* provoked an uproar. "It's a crazy idea," said Joop Atsma, a member of the ruling Dutch Christian Democratic Party, which tried to prevent it from being broadcast.[1] But the show went on.

It turned out to be a brilliant hoax. Toward the end of the program, as Lisa was about to announce her choice, the producer interrupted and revealed to the audience that she was really an actress, not a cancer patient looking for a worthy organ recipient. Lisa and the three "contestants"—all real people in need of kidney transplants and aware of the subterfuge—were part of an enactment to dramatize the desperate shortage of transplantable organs.

Yes, the televised ploy was tasteless, even shocking. Yet sensationalism has its merits—and, in this case, it called attention to the hundreds of thousands of needless deaths occurring all over the world as a result of the shortage of transplantable organs. One of the victims was Bart de Graaff, the founder of the host television network, who died in 2002 at the age of thirty-five because he could not survive the years-long wait for a new kidney. The show was meant as a tribute to him.

"We have only done this cry for help because we want to solve a problem that shouldn't be a problem," a producer told a news conference after the

1

reality show.[2] The woeful lack of organs for transplantation is a problem all over the world, and the painful reality of needless death translates into all languages.

Death and Suffering Mount

In the fall of 2008 in the United States, over 100,000 Americans were candidates for transplantable kidneys, livers, hearts, and lungs. Kidneys and partial livers may come from living donors; the rest must come from the newly deceased. Transplant candidates wait on a list maintained by the United Network for Organ Sharing (UNOS), an entity that manages the procurement and distribution of cadaver organs under monopoly contract with the federal government.

The majority of transplant candidates—three-quarters—need kidneys.[3] The high demand for kidneys reflects the fact that renal failure is the only form of vital organ collapse for which a long-term therapy is both available and sustainable for years: dialysis. During dialysis, the patient's blood is circulated through a machine that extracts toxins, maintains chemical balance, and siphons off accumulated fluid. The typical dialysis session lasts three to four hours and takes place three times a week. Most patients find it a vast intrusion into their daily lives and are often left exhausted and weakened by the process; little more than one-tenth of all individuals on dialysis are employed full or part time.[4] Because it accelerates the progression of cardiovascular disease, each additional year a patient is on dialysis means that post-transplant results will be significantly poorer.[5]

The prospects for people needing kidney transplants get dimmer each year. Twenty-five years ago, the average wait for a deceased-donor kidney in the United States was about one year; currently, the average wait is approaching five years, and, in many parts of the country, it is nearing ten.[6] Last year, over four thousand wait-listed individuals died.[7] Just as worrisome, the number of listed patients deemed ineligible to receive a kidney transplant—mostly because their conditions deteriorated while they were waiting—now accounts for one-third of all renal transplant candidates.[8]

Based on recent patterns, about one in four of the more than seventy-six thousand people currently waiting for kidneys will receive them within a year. The rest will languish while their names crawl to the top of the waiting list—an ordeal that can take five to eight years in big cities. Each day, eleven people will die because the delay was intolerable. Tragically, these people were healthy enough to benefit from a renal transplant when they were first listed. By 2010, according to a much-cited estimate, the average waiting time will be ten years for the entire country, exceeding the expected life spans of well over half of all wait-listed candidates.[9]

And the waiting list will only continue to grow. The two most prevalent causes of renal failure, type II diabetes and hypertension, become more common with age. With the baby boomers aging and the ranks of the elderly growing, new cases of end-stage renal disease will continue to appear, even if progress is made in preventing these conditions.[10] Moreover, the waiting list doesn't even reflect the full scope of the problem. A 2008 study estimates that over 130,000 dialysis patients with a "good prognosis" (that is, an expected survival of five years or longer on dialysis) are never even referred for transplantation.[11] These voiceless thousands don't show up on anybody's "list."

In this climate of scarcity, it is no surprise that desperate patients try to find organs on their own. They rent billboards and place ads in newsletters soliciting donors, join online matching sites to find willing "good Samaritan" donors, and impose upon ambivalent relatives. Some of them—no one truly knows how many—go abroad, with the sickening knowledge that their new organs might come from impoverished inhabitants of the Third World or executed prisoners in China.

This dire picture needs to change.

Altruism Isn't Enough

The metaphorical bedrock of the American transplant system is altruistic giving. Organ donation, we are told, should be the ultimate gift: the "gift of life," a sublime act of generosity. Givers must not expect (or, in the case of deceased donors, their survivors must not expect) to be enriched in any way. This is lovely sentiment, to be sure, but it is terribly inadequate as the basis for transplant policy—a reality that was first appreciated in the 1970s.[12]

Our transplant policy was established in 1984 with the passage of the National Organ Transplant Act (NOTA). The act established the Organ Procurement and Transplantation Network (OPTN) under the U.S. Department of Health and Human Services. The network then contracted with UNOS to manage all aspects of cadaver-organ procurement and distribution, including maintenance of the waiting list.

When NOTA was introduced in July 1983, spearheaded by then-Congressman Albert Gore Jr., it was silent on the question of organ sales. That matter came to national attention in September, when the *Washington Post* reported that a local physician, H. Barry Jacobs, intended to bring indigent foreigners to this country and pay each to relinquish a kidney.[13] In the fall of 1983, Jacobs presented his plan in testimony before a U.S. House of Representatives hearing on NOTA.[14] Dismayed by his cavalier style—especially when he touted the profit-making aspect of his proposal—and disturbed by the prospect of the wealthy benefiting from the desperation of the poor, the drafters of NOTA added section 301, which reads:

> **(a) Prohibition.** It shall be unlawful for any person to knowingly acquire, receive, or otherwise transfer any human organ for valuable consideration for use in human transplantation if the transfer affects interstate commerce.

> **(b) Penalties.** Any person who violates subsection (a) of this section shall be fined not more than $50,000 or imprisoned not more than five years, or both.[15]

The point was to outlaw commercialization, organ brokering, and private sales between individuals. It did not specifically bar government action to encourage organ donation through incentives. Since the passage of NOTA, the transplant establishment has become deeply committed to the idea that an organ should be a selfless gift, and that the donor must have no expectation of reward. Long forgotten is Gore's recommendation that incentives should be considered if, in the future, a system based on volunteers did not yield adequate numbers of organs.[16] Altruism is unquestionably a beautiful virtue, but it hasn't inspired enough people to donate their organs, in death or in life.

The Advantages of Living Donors

Living donation, as opposed to harvesting organs from the recently deceased, offers the greatest promise for remedying the organ shortage. For one thing, the living represent a population capable of providing a far greater volume of kidneys than the dead. Of the roughly 2 million Americans who die annually, relatively few possess organs healthy enough for transplanting. The number is estimated to range between 10,500 and 13,000, representing less than 1 percent of all deaths each year.[17] Moreover, when unaware of the preference of their loved ones, only about half of families give permission for the organs to be retrieved at death. The number of deceased donors in 2007—7,241—is consistent with these realities.[18] (Incidentally, this built-in constraint on the number of potentially transplantable kidneys underscores the reason a "presumed-consent" law—a policy in which all individuals are presumed to be organ donors at death unless they explicitly indicated otherwise while living—is unlikely to yield a huge windfall of transplantable kidneys.)[19]

Some experts suggest increasing the supply of deceased-donor organs by redefining the criteria by which people are declared dead. Currently, the vast majority of deceased donors are declared dead by brain-death criteria. However, organs have also been successfully transplanted from so-called cardiac-death donors whose critical illness has led to a decision to withdraw aggressive life-sustaining measures.[20] Many transplant experts are now urging greater reliance on organs from those who die of cardiac arrest. Given that more people die because their hearts stop than because of brain damage, it is reasonable to broaden eligibility in this way. Yet there is little reason to believe that adding these donors will significantly reduce the shortage. In 2006, the last year for which complete data exist, 1,016 kidneys were obtained from 645 donors via this procedure; as of November 2007, 1,086 kidneys were provided by 736 such donors.[21]

Besides being much more plentiful, living-donor kidneys are of better quality and greater longevity than those from the deceased. The fact that kidneys from living donors survive twice as long means fewer repeat transplants per patient and less chance of returning to dialysis.[22] In addition, a greater supply of kidneys may enable some patients with impending renal failure to avoid dialysis altogether. This is ideal, because a living-donor kidney transplanted before the recipient ever needs dialysis confers the greatest advantage of all: Not only does the organ last longer, but so does the recipient, who is spared the cardiovascular stress of dialysis. Finally, with the care of dialysis patients costing Medicare roughly $20 billion a year, considerable savings could be accrued by liberating patients sooner from the treatment or allowing them to avoid it altogether.[23]

Clearly, the advantages of living-donor kidneys for transplantation are considerable. Unfortunately, the number of cases in which these benefits may be conferred is far too few, as people are not exactly lining up to give their organs, even to patients they know and love. In 2007, only about one in nine candidates for transplants received a kidney from a family member or friend.[24] Donor compensation may be the only way to bring about a significant increase in the number of individuals—family members, friends, and, especially, strangers—who are willing to give up their own kidneys to save lives.

Compensation for Living Kidney Donors

A reconsideration of the ban imposed by the National Organ Transplant Act on offering "valuable consideration" to people in exchange for donating organs is long overdue. In this book we argue that governments—federal and state—should be allowed to motivate individuals to donate kidneys in this manner. This is the first book dedicated in a practical way to changing transplant policy to permit compensation of living donors. It describes in detail how a feasible compensation-based system could be designed, and it sets the stage for revision of the law by showing how donor rewards are ethically permissible, economically warranted, and pragmatically achievable.

The chapters ahead explore key elements of the debate surrounding the use of incentives to motivate living kidney donation. We begin by exploring the fundamental practical questions raised by transplantation: Is it safe for donors and recipients? Is it cost-effective? What could a donor compensation system look like?

In chapter 1, transplant surgeon Arthur Matas addresses the question of medical risks to living kidney donors. Reasserting the overall safety of the procedure is relevant in light of ethical concerns that donor risk is only acceptable when a preexisting emotional bond exists between provider and recipient, especially since these concerns appear to be based on the mistaken view that the risk is considerable.[25]

Next, health economist Elbert Huang and his colleagues examine the cost-effectiveness of renal transplantation. Their comprehensive analysis of previously published studies reveals the significant economic advantage of transplantation over chronic dialysis maintenance and alleviates concerns that increasing the number of transplants through donor compensation will impose a financial burden on Medicare. Savings are sustained even after taking into account the costs of rewarding donors and the ongoing medical expenditures associated with transplantation itself.

In their proposed blueprint for a compensation system, transplant surgeon David Cronin and economist Julio Elías bring together in chapter 3 the conclusions of the first three chapters. The authors outline logistics for recruiting and evaluating donors in a manner that provides for the best possible medical outcome while ensuring the donors' well-being, and for providing post-transplant medical follow-up. They also address the question of assigning economic values to incentives and outline possible types of compensation.

The book turns next to the ethical and theoretical concerns regarding incentives for donation.

The most important arguments against providing compensation to donors focus on the troubling claim that it will be impossible to implement incentive programs in an ethical manner, and to protect prospective donors from exploitation. In chapter 4, philosophers James Stacey Taylor and Mary Simmerling explain how the morally reprehensible features of overseas black markets would be prevented from emerging in a regulated and tightly supervised program in the United States. If anything, they point out, the depredations of the underground market affirm the need to test a legal mode of donor compensation.

In chapter 5, I explore the contention that donor compensation represents a taboo form of commodification and is thus an affront to human dignity. I argue that this is too narrow a moral view of transactions, and that dignity can be preserved when donors' safety is protected and they are treated with respect and gratitude. I conclude that refusing to experiment with incentives is itself an unethical posture because it perpetuates needless suffering and death.

Legal scholar Richard Epstein elaborates in chapter 6 upon the philosophical and economic weaknesses of the current regime of enforced altruism. He examines the inconsistent attitudes toward altruism within the transplant establishment, gives some estimate of net social gains that can be expected from allowing transactions, and critiques the claim that financial incentives are self-defeating.

Chapter 7 addresses another concern frequently voiced by opponents of donor compensation: that altruistic individuals would be dismayed by the commercial nature of organ-giving and thus refrain from donating, and that such refusals to donate would occur in numbers sufficient to cause the total supply of transplantable kidneys to decline. Nephrologist Benjamin Hippen and I review the relevant literature and conclude that a net reduction in transplantable kidneys is not a likely consequence of donor compensation.

In the last chapter, legal scholar Michele Goodwin takes up the question of legislative action to permit compensation for organ donors. She argues that compensation programs are best conducted at the level of the state, rather than through a more centralized arrangement. Revising NOTA to permit the U.S. Department of Health and Human Services to grant state waivers to the ban would enable states to experiment with different models of recruitment and compensation.

In the book's conclusion, I summarize the rhetorical and political forces that bear on prospective legislative change and advocate a specific policy direction and legal remedy.

Finally, four appendices at the end of the book provide further information pertinent to the issue of organ donor compensation. In appendix A, Chad Thompson presents a brief history of legislation pertaining to organ transplants. Appendix B provides a chronology of milestones in the American public's growing awareness of the organ shortage and of compensation as a means to addressing it, while appendix C reviews attitudes toward donor compensation and related questions from the perspective of public opinion polls. Appendix D gives an overview of the positions of major religions on these questions.

Calling on Congress

Offering compensation to potential organ donors is a controversial proposition. Yet, as death and suffering among kidney patients mount, physicians, legal scholars, and ethicists alike are urging pilot studies of a regulated compensation-based system with strong donor protections. This would require Congress to amend the 1984 National Organ Transplant Act so that people who provide organs to strangers could receive "valuable consideration."

It is crucial to remember that the ban on compensating donors was put in place by Congress over twenty years ago. Even in 1983, though, Representative Gore recognized that the prohibition his legislation was imposing might not serve the country's needs in the future. His acknowledgment that incentives might one day be necessary to address the organ shortage is critical to informed debate. It shows that the altruistic principle—stubbornly regarded by influential entities such as the National Kidney Foundation as the only valid motive for giving an organ—was never intended to be a fixed, sacrosanct element of transplant policy. The ban against compensation was inserted in expedient good faith, but just as Congress established the ban, it can revoke it. The law could be amended, for example, to decriminalize incentives offered by federal or state governments. Incentives at these levels could take many forms, perhaps as simple as an offer of lifelong Medicare coverage or a credit on the federal income tax. States could, perhaps, implement their own creative incentive ideas, such as the utilization of tuition vouchers, state income tax credit, loan forgiveness, or contributions to retirement accounts. The possibilities are many.

The altruistic motive is deeply noble and loving. But reliance upon it as the sole legitimate reason for giving an organ is the cause of too many unnecessary deaths. There is strong reason to believe that a compensation-based system will increase the numbers of transplantable kidneys and thus reduce needless suffering and death. This book suggests ways that such a system could be structured and explains why there is moral imperative to innovate.

1

Risks of Kidney Transplantation to a Living Donor

Arthur J. Matas

The organ donor shortage is one of the most troubling issues in kidney transplantation today. People with kidney failure live longer and better lives with transplants than they do on dialysis—the only other treatment that can keep them alive[1]—and a transplant from a living donor provides a better outcome than one from a deceased donor, especially if performed before the recipient starts dialysis.[2] Yet for many kidney transplant candidates, no living donors are available. Each year many more patients go on the transplant waiting list than undergo transplants,[3] and the waiting list, the waiting time, and the number of deaths that occur while waiting continue to grow. Currently, the median waiting time for a deceased-donor kidney is over five years.[4] For a patient with end-stage renal disease (ESRD), a form of kidney failure so severe that it is irreversible, a five-year wait is a calamity. In 2001, the annual mortality rate for prospective transplant recipients was reported to be 6.3 percent;[5] by 2005, it had increased to 8.1 percent.[6]

To be eligible to donate a kidney, a prospective living donor must meet three basic criteria. First, to minimize the possibility of the intended recipient's body rejecting the transplant, the blood type and tissue antigens of the two individuals must be compatible.[7] Second, the would-be donor must be healthy enough to undergo major surgery; and, third, the donor must have two healthy kidneys, as the remaining one will have to compensate for the loss of the donated one. Removal of the kidney takes between two and four hours, and the donor typically leaves the hospital after two or three nights. Barring complications, a donor with a desk job will generally be back at work within three to four weeks; those with more physically demanding jobs will take longer to recover sufficiently for full-time work.[8]

This is a great deal to ask of an individual, especially since living organ donation is virtually the only surgical operation with no planned benefit for the donor. In addition, the kidney removal procedure (called nephrectomy) carries an array of potential health risks. While transplant experts currently recommend donations with the understanding that the surgical risk is small and the long-term risk of living with only one kidney minimal, the ethical question of balancing the risk to the donor with the benefit to the recipient has been the subject of much debate. Defining these risks, therefore, is a prerequisite for any discussion about living donation, particularly one as fraught with controversy as that concerning donor compensation.

The undertaking is not a simple one, as evidence about risks can be hard to come by, and the field is constantly changing. Because the living kidney donor does not need the surgery for his or her physical benefit, for example, many transplant personnel historically have felt that one death in thousands of operations is excessive and have discouraged living donation. Many programs have begun only within the past ten years to recommend the procedure in response to the tremendous shortage of organs. Moreover, the shortage has also led to a relaxing of the criteria for organ donation, allowing the acceptance as donors of obese individuals and those with mildly elevated blood pressure, among others in less than perfect health—a change that complicates the task of defining the risks by altering them.

Another transition has been that from an open operation, which involves making an eight- to twelve-inch incision along the donor's flank to attain a direct view of the kidney, to a laparoscopic procedure, in which the kidney is removed through a relatively small incision on the abdomen with the aid of a camera. Since the laparoscopic procedure is less painful than the conventional one and recovery is faster, it has since the early 2000s become the procedure of choice at many transplant centers. Yet, for the most part, the operative and short-term risks have only been studied for open nephrectomy, and then only in an "ideal" donor population, leaving the actual risks of donating largely uncertain under current conditions.

The objective in this chapter, then, is to determine the risks of living kidney donation, based on the evidence available, in terms of the surgery, the perioperative period of several weeks following it, and the long-term consequences, if any, of the procedure, with particular attention paid to cases of laparoscopic nephrectomy and less-stringent donor criteria.

Surgical and Perioperative Risks

The biggest risk of removing a kidney from a living donor is the surgery itself. For two decades, the rate of perioperative mortality (death within thirty days after surgery) has been reported to be 3 in 10,000 (0.03 percent) in studies that have included, among others, two national surveys of transplant centers—the first conducted in 1991, the second in 2002.[9] In the 2002 survey, which examined a similar number of open and laparoscopic nephrectomies, all three of the donor deaths occurred after laparoscopic surgery; so for a study published in 2006, Friedman and colleagues canvassed members of the American Society of Transplant Surgeons by mail and asked about complications associated specifically with the laparoscopic technique. They reported two donor deaths from hemorrhage (massive bleeding) and two incidents of shock. Unfortunately, the report failed to include the number of operations performed, and without this denominator, it is difficult to interpret these results. Moreover, the survey completion rate of only 22 percent was low.[10]

Nonfatal complications can also occur in living donors in the days following surgery. The once-standard open nephrectomy has been associated with major complication rates, involving extended hospital stays or second operations to correct problems, of 1 to 2 percent. These complications include reversible problems such as wound infection, bleeding, urinary tract infection, or incisional hernia.[11] Although the 2002 survey of transplant centers found a higher rate of complications and reoperations in laparoscopic donors than in open donors, the rate for laparoscopic donors was still relatively low; second operations were necessary in only 0.9 percent, and the rate of complications not requiring reoperation was the same. The survey data may, moreover, have overstated the rate of complications because the time period covered included only the early experience with laparoscopic nephrectomy at many centers. As with many new surgical procedures, laparoscopic nephrectomy is associated with a learning curve for both center and surgeon at first. Su and colleagues reported a significant decrease in laparoscopic donor complications over time at their institution.[12]

While laparoscopic nephrectomy is associated with markedly less blood loss, shorter hospital stays, less need for narcotics, earlier resumption of normal diets, and faster return to normal activities[13] than open nephrectomy,[14] any kidney removal is a major operation requiring the patient to spend significant time under anesthesia. Since the kidney is directly attached to two of the major blood vessels,[15] the risk of complications and even death persists. Also to be taken into account is the fact that, until recently, only perfectly healthy living donors were accepted at most transplant centers, and so reports of both mortality and complications were based on individuals who were thoroughly screened and in impeccable health. The current use of expanded-criteria donors may be increasing both short-term and long-term risks.

Long-Term Outcome

In addition to carrying surgical and perioperative risks, removal of one kidney may have a long-term impact on donor survival time and on the function of the remaining kidney, as the result either of the surgery itself or the loss of the added physiological "buffer" provided by two healthy kidneys. What does the research tell us about these outcomes?

Survival Time. It is difficult to draw conclusions about long-term survival for kidney donors because living-donor transplants have been done routinely for only a relatively short time, not beginning in earnest at many centers until the early 1980s. Furthermore, follow-up studies differ widely in terms of the ages of the donors, which range from eighteen to sixty-five years; this makes it difficult to find the proper comparison group of non-donors. A few studies have had telling results, however.

A decade ago in Sweden, for example, Fehrman-Ekholm and colleagues found that living kidney donors actually lived longer than those of similar age in the general nondonor population.[16] There was some selection bias in the Fehrman-Ekholm finding—that is, a bias built into the study by the choice of subjects—since donors tend to be healthier than the average individual, and healthier people tend to live longer. Nonetheless, the study—at the minimum—suggested that removal of a single kidney does not shorten life.

Much can also be learned from studies of patients who have had one kidney removed for reasons unrelated to transplant surgery. Andersen and others compared the survival rates of 232 nondonor patients who had undergone nephrectomy for benign disease with the Danish population from which they were drawn. Follow-up time ranged from two months to twenty-six years. The researchers found that if the remaining kidney was normal, the patients' survival time was identical to that of the overall population.[17]

Finally, a number of studies have found that in the general nondonor population, patients with mild abnormalities in renal function have a higher rate of cardiovascular disease even when they have two kidneys.[18] This is of some concern, because such abnormalities are not uncommon after kidney donation. Kidney donors have thus far not been found to be at any increased risk for cardiovascular disease, however. Perhaps kidney removal is not associated with sufficient renal dysfunction to increase the risk for cardiovascular disease, or perhaps we have not followed donors long enough to be able to discern any increased risk. Additional long-term studies are needed to resolve this issue.

Renal Function Twenty or More Years after Donation. Numerous studies have compared renal function and other health indicators in donors before and after surgery.[19] Immediately after removal of one kidney there is a loss of 50 percent of renal function, but the remaining kidney quickly starts to compensate. Within seven days after donation, measures of kidney function increase to 70 percent of presurgery levels; by six weeks, they rise to nearly 80 percent.[20]

Studies have shown no significant long-term consequences of living kidney donation. Although isolated cases of renal failure after kidney removal have been reported,[21] no study that has followed a large number of donors has found any evidence of progressive deterioration. In recognition of the very low risks, most insurance companies do not even increase premiums for kidney donors.[22] A limiting factor in most of these studies, however, is that the average follow-up time has been less than twenty years. Since most living donors have a life expectancy of more than twenty years, longer follow-up is necessary for a complete analysis of the risks.[23]

Four published studies do provide this longer follow-up. A 1992 University of Minnesota study compared the transplant center's own living donors with their nondonor siblings.[24] Of the 130 people who donated kidneys between January 1963 and December 1970, data were obtained on 78.[25] Of these, 15 had died two to twenty-five years after donation, but none of them had kidney disease at death.

For the 57 surviving donors who completed laboratory testing, all measures of kidney function observed in the study[26] were within the normal ranges; and although about one-third were taking drugs for high blood pressure and about 0.25 percent had proteinuria (protein in the urine, which is sometimes a sign of kidney disease), the donors' siblings did not differ significantly from them on the major characteristics of interest.[27] This suggests that medical conditions developing sometime after donation were likely to occur in these donors even if they had not given their kidneys.

About a decade after this study, the Minnesota team conducted a similar one, reviewing its living donors who underwent nephrectomy between June 1963 and December 1979 and bringing the maximum follow-up span to thirty-seven years.[28] Out of a total of 773 donors, data were obtained on 380 who were alive more than twenty years after donation.[29] Of these, three had abnormal kidney function, and two had undergone transplantation. The other 375 all had normal kidney function, and their rates of proteinuria and hypertension were similar to those of people of similar age in the general population. Among the patients who had died before the investigators could revisit their medical status—eighty-four in all—three had been on dialysis at the time of death, but their deaths were largely attributable to other diseases.[30]

A third study by Goldfarb and colleagues followed living donors twenty to thirty-two years after nephrectomy.[31] Of 180 eligible subjects, 70 (39 percent) participated in the study. For them, serum creatinine levels (a rise in which is indicative of renal dysfunction) and blood pressure were higher than the predonation levels; all values were, however, still within the normal ranges. Proteinuria was reported in thirteen (19 percent) of the seventy, and two developed renal failure requiring dialysis. The overall incidence of high blood pressure was comparable to that among people of similar age in the nondonor population.

A fourth follow-up investigation—the study by Fehrman-Ekholm and others already mentioned—surveyed 1,112 donors who underwent nephrectomy in Goteborg, Sweden.[32] Of these, six (0.5 percent) developed renal failure fourteen to twenty-seven years after donation. In one of the six (a donor forty-five years of age), cancer developed in the remaining kidney, which then had to be removed. The other five donors were seventy-three to eighty-three years old at the time their end-stage disease was diagnosed. The investigators calculated the expected rate of renal failure in people of similar age in Sweden's nondonor population and concluded that kidney donors suffered no increase in this outcome.

Future Concerns. In the United States, a growing epidemic of high blood pressure and adult-onset diabetes—both due, partly, to a rising wave of obesity—predisposes individuals to higher risk of kidney failure.[33] Similarly, both obesity and smoking have recently been associated with the development of proteinuria.[34] In one study of nondonors who had kidneys removed for reasons other than transplantation, the probability of proteinuria was 60 percent in obese patients[35] ten years after their surgery, rising to 92 percent after twenty years. In contrast, the probability of proteinuria ten years after surgery for patients who were not obese was a mere 7 percent; after twenty years, it was still only 23 percent.[36] Given that obese individuals are now accepted as kidney donors, these findings are of some concern. Additional studies are necessary to determine if this type of donor is subject to increased long-term risk.

Comparative Progress of Kidney Disease. A critical question which so far has been very little explored is whether living donors who subsequently develop any form of kidney disease, even years after nephrectomy, will experience renal failure more quickly than nondonors with kidney disease. A long-term donor follow-up study published in 2002 by the University of Minnesota researchers identified nineteen living donors who developed diabetes six to thirty-four years after donation.[37] In addition, a small number of nondonors with diabetes or with polycystic kidney disease (a hereditary condition in which both kidneys develop multiple, enlarging cysts) who underwent nephrectomy were studied.[38] The limited evidence suggests they did not develop renal failure more rapidly than patients with those same diseases who had not undergone nephrectomy.

Quality of Life. In general, living kidney donors report a quality of life similar to, or even better than, that of people in the general population.[39] Some concerns have been raised, however, about recovery and future health,[40] the amount of time taken to return to routine daily activities and commitments,[41] financial consequences,[42] and potential penalization by life or health insurance companies following kidney donation.[43] In addition, many living donors report feeling abandoned by the transplant program after surgery and are disappointed by the lack of follow-up after their discharge from the hospital.[44]

All of these findings warrant further investigation. Because most living donors to date have been relatives of the recipients, most studies have been of living related donors, which leaves questions concerning unrelated donors. Most, moreover, have involved donors who underwent open nephrectomy. Anecdotal reports suggest that the problem of poor to nonexistent follow-up besets laparoscopic donors, too.[45] Learning if the same issues develop for unrelated donors and after laparoscopic nephrectomy will be important to designing protocols for transplant programs that increase satisfaction with the process for all living donors.

Conclusion

Obtaining comprehensive answers to questions about risks to living kidney donors is critical, especially with regard to long-term follow-up. Since many donors are in their twenties and thirties at the time of donation, it is important to understand any increased risks four, or even six, decades later. The National Institutes of Health recently provided funding to a consortium of transplant centers to study long-term donor risks. The goal of the consortium is to obtain follow-up information on all donors from the 1960s, 1970s, and 1980s. Research on surgical and perioperative risks will doubtless continue, as well.

In the meantime, what conclusions should be drawn about the risks of living kidney donation by individuals who are considering becoming donors? First, they must appreciate that donation is major surgery and, like any major surgery, it carries real, though low, risks of serious complications and, rarely, death. Recuperation from laparoscopic surgery is relatively rapid, with several weeks to resumption of most tasks (except for heavy physical exertion). Second, they should know that, following surgery, donors live longer than the general population. This makes sense as they are, in general, a very healthy population to begin with. Also, the overall mental and physical health of donors is comparable to that of the general population; where there are differences, they have manifested as slightly higher rates of elevated blood pressure and above-average levels of protein in the urine. There is no evidence that these differences contribute to future medical problems for the donor.

In terms of our understanding of long-term outcome for living donors, the retrospective nature of the studies so far conducted, the relatively small number of living donors studied, and the often low response rates to donor questionnaires constitute major limitations. Also, no study to date has been able to obtain long-term follow-up data on every patient in its sample. Still, no study has shown an increased rate of mortality or complications, including renal disease, among donors who, it must be emphasized, are healthy people to begin with. Long-term quality of life, moreover, appears to be excellent after donation.

2

The Cost-Effectiveness of Renal Transplantation

Elbert S. Huang, Nidhi Thakur, and David O. Meltzer

The outlook for patients diagnosed with chronic renal failure improved dramatically in 1972, when Congress mandated the establishment of the End Stage Renal Disease (ESRD) Program under the umbrella of Medicare. This program was created to provide dialysis and kidney transplantation for renal patients regardless of age, income, disability level, or insurance coverage, as long as they were legitimate beneficiaries of Social Security.

Whereas patients with end-stage renal disease were almost certain to face premature death before the ESRD program was established, after 1972 the number of patients living with chronic renal failure rose sharply and steadily. Early studies predicted that 10,000 new patients would begin dialysis each year, an estimate that later proved to be a vast underestimate of the actual growth in the dialysis population.[1] In 1978, for example, over 14,000 new patients initiated dialysis; in 1986, this number had grown to 32,000.[2] By 2005, there were 97,143 patients beginning dialysis, and the total number of dialysis patients had reached 314,000.[3]

In tandem with the rising number of patients, annual dialysis expenditures quickly ballooned. The first year of implementation required a budget of $229 million, with the expectation that costs would level off at about $250 million per year.[4] With the successful treatment of thousands of new patients, expenditures instead rose exponentially: $1.4 billion was spent in 1980; $3 billion in 1987; $5 billion in 1990; and $12.3 billion in 1998.[5] Given that this figure had increased to $17 billion per year by 2005,[6] a

on to the federal government by 2010 is not
D participants, who represented 1.2 percent
ccounted for 8.2 percent of the Medicare
; same subgroup was responsible for only

ay a dialysis patient can cease treatment is
.....ssiul organ transplant; yet over 130,000 dialysis patients
with a "good prognosis" (defined as an expected survival of five years or
longer on dialysis) are never even referred for transplantation.[10] In addition
to conferring great clinical benefits, an increased transplantation rate would
translate to considerable cost-savings in ESRD treatment. In the following
discussion we will show that renal transplantation has been repeatedly
found to reduce health-care costs significantly in comparison with dialysis,
with transplant recipients experiencing improved health both in terms of
additional years and quality of life. These findings have been consistent over
three decades and across nations, and they suggest that the added cost of
compensation for kidney donors would not make transplantation less cost-
effective in comparison with dialysis, even if the cost difference between the
two treatments were smaller than they currently are.

Economic Studies of Renal Replacement Therapy

The costs of ESRD are, in large part, directly attributable to routine renal
replacement therapy (RRT), which is necessary for all ESRD patients to
remain alive. RRT options include hemodialysis, peritoneal dialysis, and
renal (kidney) transplantation. Hemodialysis is the regular removal of waste
products from the blood, for which patients are attached to a machine by
some form of intravenous access. Patients typically have hemodialysis sessions lasting three to four hours, three days per week, at outpatient facilities.
Peritoneal dialysis is the regular removal of waste products by the placement
of specially formulated fluids into the abdominal cavity. Peritoneal dialysis
must be performed on a daily basis, but can be done at home. Renal transplantation is the replacement of the patient's poorly functioning kidneys by
a kidney from a deceased or living donor. Successful transplantation elimi-
nates the need for dialysis but requires the patient to take a regular regimen

of immunosuppressive medications for the remainder of his or her life to help prevent the recipient's own immune system from attacking and rejecting the new kidney.

Of the several types of renal replacement therapies, transplantation is the most clinically effective. According to life expectancy figures from 2005, a man between the ages of forty and forty-four could expect to live just over eight years on dialysis; if he were to receive a transplant, he could expect to live just over twenty-three more years than that. Drawing on these same figures, a woman between fifty-five and fifty-nine could expect to live just over five years on dialysis, and very nearly an additional sixteen years with a transplant.[11] In addition, an individual's quality of life would improve dramatically once he or she were no longer dependent on dialysis in any form.[12]

The various forms of renal replacement therapy are some of the most frequently studied treatments in the health economics literature, in part because of the substantial health and economic burdens of ESRD. One of the principal purposes of economic evaluations of health-care technologies such as RRT is to quantify the relative value of various treatment or diagnostic options in order to set priorities for the allocation of scarce resources.[13] Economic studies of RRT have been conducted using both cost-benefit analysis and cost-effectiveness analysis. Cost-benefit analysis enumerates costs and benefits of a program in dollars or other currency units.[14] In the health-care context, this requires assigning a monetary value to the length and quality of life. Because this explicit evaluation of outcomes has made cost-benefit analysis controversial from an ethical perspective, cost-effectiveness analysis has been more commonly used for economic evaluation in health care.

In cost-effectiveness analysis, the costs and health benefits of alternative medical interventions are compared from a societal perspective.[15] This allows scholars to determine the *incremental cost-effectiveness ratio* (ICER) between two or more medical practices or policies—that is, the incremental cost per unit of health gained with one treatment program compared to another. In the current health-care environment, it is rare for a patient with a given condition to go without any treatment, and so the relevant comparator for a treatment in a cost-effectiveness analysis is usually an alternative treatment as opposed to no treatment at all.

When comparing two treatments, the ICER can be expressed with the formula

$$\frac{(Cost_2 - Cost_1)}{(Effectiveness_2 - Effectiveness_1)}$$

The difference in costs between two treatments includes, at minimum, differences in the direct medical costs of caring for patients, such as the costs of medications, diagnostic tests, procedures, and hospitalizations, and also indirect costs, such as the time devoted by patients and caregivers to carrying out treatment plans. A societal perspective on costs should also include all future net resources used (nonmedical consumption plus medical expenditure minus earnings).[16] Differences in the effectiveness of treatments can be expressed using different measurements, including the rate of specific complications, life expectancy or life years, and quality-adjusted life years (QALYs). The QALY is intended to account for changes in both morbidity and mortality, and analyses that use the QALY as a measure of effectiveness are referred to as cost-utility analyses. QALYs are calculated by multiplying the time spent in specific health states by quality-of-life weights called utilities that are assigned to those specific health states.[17] An alternative to the quality-adjusted life year is the disability-adjusted life year (DALY), a measure that accounts for morbidity in terms of disability rather than quality of life.[18]

The ICER that is generated by a cost-effectiveness analysis must be interpreted with specific attention to the magnitude and direction of the difference in costs (the numerator in the above formula) and the difference in effectiveness (the denominator). In cases where the difference in effectiveness is negative, the treatment in question is harmful in comparison to another and would therefore not be considered as a desirable alternative (unless it actually saved money, in which case the more costly and effective baseline treatment option might be better viewed as the treatment whose cost-effectiveness was being considered). In cases where the effectiveness measure is positive, the treatment in question improves the health of patients, or is beneficial. Such a treatment would therefore be considered for adoption.

Among treatments that are beneficial, some are cost-saving compared to the alternative, while others incur additional expense. Beneficial cost-saving treatments are, unfortunately, rare, since the majority of new treatments improve health but at an additional expense. Whether a given additional expense for better health is worthwhile is often the subject of intense debate and controversy, especially in relation to insurance coverage decisions. ICER results for new treatments are typically compared to historical ICER thresholds for treatments that are already reimbursed by government or private insurers.

Because medical coverage of patients with ESRD is explicitly covered by federal mandate, the ICERs from cost-effectiveness analyses of renal replacement therapy have been used as thresholds for subsequent analyses of other therapies in all areas of medical cost-effectiveness analysis. The threshold most commonly used in determining if a treatment is worthwhile is $50,000 per life year gained.[19] Many have criticized the appropriateness of this threshold, which actually comes from a Canadian study of the cost-effectiveness of hemodialysis, and more recent studies of the value of health improvements have suggested thresholds of $100,000 to $400,000 per life year gained, with midpoint estimates most often around $200,000.[20] These thresholds are used to assess ICERs generated from cost-effectiveness analyses of new treatment interventions; those with ICERs lower than the thresholds are considered to be of good value.

Gathering the Data

To assemble an overall picture of the cost-effectiveness of kidney transplants as compared to other renal replacement therapies, we searched a number of electronic databases, including the Harvard/Tufts database of cost-effectiveness analysis (CEA) studies, the Cochrane Library of CEA studies, and the MEDLINE for studies published from 1968 to 2007, using the key words "kidney transplantation" and "cost-effectiveness" or "renal transplantation" and "cost-effectiveness." In addition, we checked the references of initially identified studies, as well as those included in a recently conducted review article.[21] We excluded CEA studies that only evaluated the economic value of specific innovations in renal transplantation management, such as new immunosuppressive agents. Instead, we focused specifically on the overall economic value of renal transplantation.

In total, we found seventeen studies describing unique analyses assessing the cost-effectiveness of renal transplantation.[22] From each, we gathered data including year of publication, country of origin, perspective of analysis (that is, whether the cost-effectiveness of the various treatments were viewed from a societal perspective or from that of a public insurer, such as Medicare), treatment comparison, difference in costs, difference in health effects, and the incremental cost-effectiveness ratio. Our review included studies reporting the different measures of effectiveness described earlier (such as life years, quality-adjusted life years, and disability-adjusted life years), and we converted all ICERs to 2006 U.S. dollars for purposes of comparison.

Having collected all this information, we next grouped the studies by treatment comparison. As mentioned earlier, patients today rarely go without any treatment for their conditions, so the more recent studies have directly compared different forms of renal replacement therapy, namely hemodialysis and renal transplantation. The majority of early studies presented the cost-effectiveness ratio of various forms of renal replacement therapy as compared to no therapy for patients with end-stage renal disease. In both periods, some studies have done both.

Results for renal transplantation were further subdivided by type. Some studies ignored the differences in economic value between cadaveric (deceased) donor renal transplantation (CDRT) and living donor renal transplantation (LDRT). Others evaluated CDRT and LDRT separately. This latter distinction is significant, since the effectiveness of LDRT is greater than that of CDRT.

The Cost-Effectiveness of Transplantation versus No Treatment

Twelve studies provided estimates of the cost-effectiveness of renal transplantation versus no treatment for end-stage renal disease, shown in tables 2-1 and 2-2. In each of these studies, the costs and health effects of each individual form of renal replacement therapy were compared to the costs and health effects of pursuing no treatment; more precisely, renal transplantation was compared with no treatment, and then hemodialysis was compared with no treatment. These analyses, therefore, provided parallel incremental cost-effectiveness ratios for renal transplantation and for various forms of hemodialysis, allowing for an indirect comparison of transplantation and hemodialysis.

In all studies, renal transplantation had the lowest ICER, which is to say, it produced the greatest health benefit at the lowest cost per unit of benefit (see table 2-2). For example, the study by Klarman examined the cost-effectiveness of center-based hemodialysis (CHD in the table), home hemodialysis (HHD), and renal transplantation, each compared to no treatment. It found that renal transplantation produced the most cost-effective increase in life expectancy. As compared to no treatment, the ICER for center-based hemodialysis was $71,800 per life year; for home hemodialysis it was $26,000 per life year; and for renal transplantation it was $16,000 per life year.[23] In layman's terms, this means that the cost to society of a year of life from funding a kidney transplant would be $16,000, while providing the same degree of extended health through dialysis would cost $26,000 (for dialysis at home) or $71,800 (for dialysis in a hospital).

Across these twelve studies, the ICERs for renal transplantation ranged from $16,000 to $69,000 per life year gained. Between the two forms of renal transplantation, living-donor transplants (LDRT) had a consistently lower ICER than cadaveric donations (CDRT). These differences ranged from approximately $7,000 per life year to $22,000 per life year.

Cost-Effectiveness of Transplantation versus Hemodialysis

Seven studies provided data that allowed for the direct evaluation of the cost-effectiveness of renal transplantation versus hemodialysis (table 2-3). In six of the seven, renal transplantation was found to reduce costs while increasing, respectively, life years, quality-adjusted life years, or disability-adjusted life years. This finding has been consistent since 1968. Cleemput and colleagues found transplantation to be a very good value as compared to dialysis even in nonadherent patient populations—that is, among patients who only irregularly took their immunosuppressive medications following transplant.[24]

In sum, with renal transplantation consistently demonstrating greater benefits than either hemodialysis or no treatment at a ratio that compares favorably to accepted thresholds for cost-effectiveness, the literature

TABLE 2-1

COST AND EFFECTIVENESS RESULTS COMPARING DIFFERENT FORMS OF
RENAL REPLACEMENT THERAPY TO NO TREATMENT

Author and year	Country	Perspective	Renal transplantation		
			Non-specific RT		CDRT
			ΔC	ΔE	ΔC
Klarman 1968	USA	Societal	$44K	17LY	—
Stange 1978	USA	Public insurer			—
Roberts 1980	USA	Public insurer	—	—	$123K
Ludbrook 1981	United Kingdom	Societal	NA	NA	—
Schersten 1986	Sweden	Unclear			—
Garner 1987	USA	Public insurer	—	—	NA
		Societal	—	—	NA
Sesso 1990	Brazil	Public insurer	—	—	
Croxson 1990	New Zealand	Public insurer	—	—	
Karlberg 1995	Sweden	Unclear			—
Laupacis 1996	Canada	Societal	$67K (yr 1)	0.65 QALY (yr 1)	—
			$27K (yr 2)	0.62 (yr 2)	
De Wit 1998	Netherlands	Societal	NA	NA	—
Kaminota 2001†	Japan	Societal	—	—	26K Yen

NOTES: RT = renal transplantation; CDRT = cadaveric donor renal transplantation; LDRT = living donor renal transplantation; CHD = center hemodialysis; HHD = home hemodialysis; ΔC = difference in costs (as originally reported); ΔE = difference in effectiveness; NA = data not available in publication;

strongly supports the idea that renal transplantation can be a highly cost-effective therapy in the general population of persons with end-stage renal disease.

The one exception to this finding was a 2003 study by Jassal and colleagues of renal transplantation in the elderly. They found that while transplantation did improve patient health in this important subpopula-

Renal transplantation			Hemodialysis			
CDRT	LDRT		CHD		HHD	
ΔE	ΔC	ΔE	ΔC	ΔE	ΔC	ΔE
—	—	—	$104K	9LY	$38K	9LY
—	—	—				
8LY	$108K	14LY	$209K	8.4LY	$126K	9.5LY
—	—	—	NA	NA	NA	NA
—	—	—			—	—
NA	NA	NA	NA	NA	NA	NA
NA	NA	NA	NA	NA	NA	NA
					—	—
—	—	—			—	—
—	—	—	$72K	0.52 QALY	—	—
—	—	—	NA	NA	—	—
12 DALYs	26K Yen	15 DALYs	131K Yen	20 DALYs	—	—

LY = life year; QALY = quality-adjusted life year; DALY = disability-adjusted life year; † = numbers reflect average difference in costs and effectiveness for patients 0–50 years of age.

tion, the benefits came at an additional cost compared to hemodialysis. This cost per additional gain in health rose in older ages. For a cadaveric transplant with a two-year waiting period, the ICER for a healthy sixty-five-year-old was $80,731 per quality-adjusted year, while for a patient older than seventy-five it rose to $118,576 per QALY.[25] This observation of rising ICERs with advancing age is typical of many cost-effectiveness

TABLE 2-2

INCREMENTAL COST-EFFECTIVENESS RATIOS FOR STUDIES COMPARING DIFFERENT FORMS OF RENAL REPLACEMENT THERAPY TO NO TREATMENT

Author and year	Country	Perspective
Klarman 1968	USA	Societal
Stange 1978	USA	Public insurer
Roberts 1980	USA	Public insurer
Ludbrook 1981	United Kingdom	Societal
Schersten 1986	Sweden	Unclear
Garner 1987	USA	Public insurer
Garner 1987	USA	Societal
Sesso 1990	Brazil	Public insurer
Croxson 1990	New Zealand	Public insurer
Karlberg 1995	Sweden	Unclear
Laupacis 1996	Canada	Societal
De Wit 1998	Netherlands	Societal
Kaminota 2001	Japan	Societal

NOTES: ICER = incremental cost-effectiveness ratio; RT = renal transplantation; CDRT = cadaveric donor renal transplantation; LDRT = living donor renal transplantation; CHD = center hemodialysis;

analyses of preventive therapies;[26] the health gains of medical treatments are typically smaller for older patients than younger ones because of their relatively shorter life expectancy. Nevertheless, the ICERs found in this study were still well below modern thresholds for defining cost-effective therapies. In addition, the variable that was the most important determi-

| ICER (treatment compared to no treatment, 2006 U.S. dollars) | | | | |
| Renal transplantation | | | Hemodialysis | |
Non-specific RT	CDRT	LDRT	CHD	HHD
16,086/LY	—	—	71,805/LY	25,994/LY
44,762–54,670/LY	—	—	93,603/LY	59,916/LY
—	45,927/LY	23,780/LY	76,351/LY	40,915/LY
27,743–39,749/LY	—	—	60,615–95,702/LY	43,946–49,541/LY
16,436–25,761/LY	—	—	77,167/LY	—
—	49,891––68,775/LY	37,418–49,541/LY	69,707–70,640/LY	55,603–56,069/LY
—	31,357–61,314/LY	19,117–41,614/LY	61,430–70,640/LY	39,749–49,658/LY
—	13,056/LY	5,712/LY	18,767/LY	—
—	19,350/LY	—	36,952/LY	29,491/LY
13,871/LY	—	—	83,346/LY	—
110,972/ QALY (yr 1) 48,026/ QALY (yr 2)	—	—	150,605/ QALY	—
15,737/LY 17,485/QALY	—	—	83,462/LY 119,248/QALY	—
—	27,567/ DALY	21,476/ DALY	113,332/ DALY	—

HHD = home hemodialysis; LY = life year; QALY = quality-adjusted life year; DALY = disability-adjusted life year.

nant of whether transplantation would be cost-effective in elderly patients was time spent waiting for a cadaveric transplant. Transplantation in the elderly became less valuable the longer the patients waited, suggesting that living-donor transplantation may be particularly beneficial in this population.

TABLE 2-3

STUDIES COMPARING RENAL TRANSPLANTATION AND HEMODIALYSIS

Author and year	Unique question	Country	Difference in costs of RT over costs of HD (originally reported, time span)	Difference in Effectiveness of RT over HD	ICER (2006 U.S. dollars)
Klarman 1968		USA	−$59,500	8 LYs	Transplant cost-saving
Roberts 1980	—	USA	−$100,616 (LDRT)	5.57 LYs	Transplant cost-saving
Laupacis 1996	—	Canada	−$7,119 (year 1) −$43,395 (year 2)	0.12 QALY (year 1) 0.11 QALY (year2)	Transplant cost-saving
Jassal 2003	Elderly population	North America	$77,000 (lifespan for healthy 65 year-old; CDRT, 2 year wait)	1.1 QALYs	80,731/ QALY
Whiting 2004	Organ donor initiatives	Canada	−$104,000 (20 years)	1.99 QALYs	Transplant cost-saving
Matas 2003	Payment for living donor kidneys	USA	−$94,579 (20 years)	3.5 QALYs	Transplant cost-saving
Cleemput 2004	Adherence	Europe	−$48,717 Euros (adherent) −$86,897 Euros (nonadherent)	5.20 QALYs (adherent) 4.09 QALYs (nonadherent)	Transplant cost-saving

NOTES: RT = renal transplantation; HD = hemodialysis; CDRT = cadaveric donor renal transplantation; LDRT = living donor renal transplantation; LY = life year; QALY = quality-adjusted life year; DALY = disability-adjusted life year.

The Cost and Benefits of Kidney Transplantation and the Value of a Kidney

The monetary value of a kidney has rarely been considered in the numerous cost-effectiveness analyses that have been conducted of kidney transplantation, with most studies having limited their cost-accounting to the direct expenses of organ procurement and the transplant procedure. For example,

Hornberger and colleagues used Health Care Financing Administration data to estimate a cost of $64,660 for an initial transplant and $70,480 for a second transplant.[27] These estimates did not include the value of the kidney itself to the recipient, nor any of the costs (medical or nonmedical) possibly incurred by a living donor.

One approach to calculating the monetary value of a kidney is to determine how high that value would have to be to shift the overall conclusion of a cost-effectiveness analysis—in other words, to assess how much a kidney would have to cost to prevent transplantation from being more cost-effective than hemodialysis. The study by Matas and colleagues did this in its investigation of society's willingness to pay for living unrelated-donor kidneys.[28] Based on the assumption that every living-donor kidney shortens the waiting list for a cadaveric kidney, the study compared the costs of hypothetical patients' receiving living-donor kidneys versus their spending a lifetime on dialysis waiting for donors. They found that living unrelated-donor kidney transplants would be cost-saving for society if the patients paid donors up to $102,000 for their organs—a figure essentially representing the costs saved by choosing a living unrelated-donor kidney transplant over dialysis. Moreover, if one were to incorporate the value of the gain in quality-adjusted life years resulting from a living unrelated-donor kidney transplant into this estimation, transplantation would remain cost-effective even if the cost of the kidney were to rise as high as $306,403. Matas and colleagues based this calculation on a value of $50,000 per QALY. Using a higher value of a QALY would have further increased this allowable cost of transplantation.

Conclusion

Renal transplantation, especially living-donor renal transplantation, is the most beneficial treatment option for patients with end-stage renal disease and is highly cost-effective compared to no therapy. In comparison to dialysis, renal transplantation has been found to reduce costs by nontrivial amounts while improving health both in terms of the number of years of life and the quality of those years of life. These findings have been consistent over three decades and across nations.

While the studies examined here consistently indicated that renal transplantation is a good value for society, very few directly acknowledged the limited supply of available kidneys, and none acknowledged the cost of the kidney in terms of payment to a donor. We suspect that the cost of a kidney has been excluded from analyses because of the highly controversial nature of assessing such a cost.

Controversy aside, economic evaluations of transplantation programs should consider including the cost of a kidney to provide a more valid assessment of alternative programs. This is not a simple matter. To some extent, the cost of a kidney can be ascertained from its value on the current black market, but on a regulated, legal market its cost would surely be quite different. Among the studies we reviewed, only one put a price on a living kidney, placing it at approximately $300,000.[29] This value was estimated without any consideration of the interaction of market supply and demand and represents a purely intrinsic value of a live kidney. If living kidneys become more readily available, this price should eventually decrease, leaving buyers with a surplus.

As the legal and ethical debate surrounding kidney transplantation evolves, so, too, will the economic evaluation of kidney transplantation programs. Current health economic studies are increasingly evaluating efforts to increase the supply of kidneys by methods such as the use of organs from expanded-criteria donors (ECD). These kidneys, which may come from living or cadaveric donors, are typically not absolutely healthy and would be considered less than ideal. Although the risk of their failing is greater, the high value and continuing shortage of kidneys suggest that transplantation of ECD kidneys might also have the potential to be both clinically valuable and cost-effective under some circumstances.

The medical community, having now understood the cost-effectiveness of renal transplantation, has begun to address secondary health-economic questions about the procedure. A recent study examined the role of recipients' preferences in treatment decisions, including those toward accepting or rejecting a kidney based on increased information about its quality.[30] It was found that incorporating the patient preferences led to a 6 percent increase in quality-adjusted life years. Also to be considered are the economic implications of retransplantation, which Hornberger has examined. This practice is becoming more common, as patients now outlive their first transplanted kidneys.

Future medical innovations, such as retransplantation, will clearly affect the calculations presented here. The long-term economic value and impact of kidney transplantation will continue to change as, for instance, improvements in immunosuppressive medications enhance patients' ability to stave off organ rejection while minimizing side effects of the drugs. Future cost-effectiveness analyses of kidney transplantation will be needed to help establish the economic value of therapeutic innovations, revise the economic value of renal transplantation versus dialysis, and, perhaps, determine the setting of financial incentives for organ donation.

3

Operational Organization of a System for Compensated Living Organ Providers

David C. Cronin II and Julio J. Elías

In the face of the growing shortage of donor kidneys for patients critically ill with end-stage renal disease, the only feasible way to eliminate the long queues for transplants is to increase the supply of organs. Many strategies have been undertaken to accomplish this: the institution of the Breakthrough Collaborative, sponsored by the Health Resources and Services Administration (HRSA);[1] the development of donor registries; the acknowledgment of advance directives, such as donor cards and driver's license designations; the launching of awareness campaigns; and, more recently, a program focused on exchanges among multiple donors and recipients.[2] Despite modest gains, however, all these efforts have failed to narrow appreciably the gap between the supply of and demand for donor organs. In the last decade, the shortage has become so severe that many transplant experts and organizations, including the ethics committees of the United Network for Organ Sharing (UNOS), the American Medical Association, and the American Society of Transplant Surgeons, have started to reconsider programs based on donor compensation as a more effective way to encourage donations.[3]

Many initiatives to increase organ donations through payments have concentrated exclusively on organs from deceased donors. Even if we were to attain all potential deceased-donor organs, however (approximately 1–2 percent of all deaths each year result in usable organs), the current and projected demand would not be met.[4] The proposal we present here, therefore, will focus on compensating living providers.[5]

Our focus on living providers is motivated by several facts: The living provide the largest pool of potential organs for transplantation; living donors currently provide kidneys for over 40 percent of all kidney transplants; and kidneys from living donors result in the best patient- and organ-survival rates for recipients.[6] Furthermore, compensation offered directly to living providers avoids several problems that might occur with compensated deceased-donor transplants. The latter process might be complicated, for instance, by families refusing to allow the organs to be taken after death, or familial disagreement and tension over whether to accept remuneration, and to whom it should go. And while the indelicacy of offering a reward to the immediately bereaved would be averted by a forward market, in which the estate of a prospective provider would receive payment upon his death if his organs were usable, it would leave unaddressed the fact that the demand for kidneys would far outstrip the deceased-provider supply even if all usable organs were harvested.

A further constraint we have placed on our proposed system is the exclusion of the paid provision of organs by the living to specified individuals. Such directed transfers would still be permitted, but they would not be compensated. The intention is to preserve private opportunities for people driven by a sense of loving obligation to rescue their sick friends or relatives. This system of directed donors would be able to act quickly. A compensation scheme, by contrast, would be a government-sponsored mechanism by which distribution of organs to a waiting population of candidates would be driven without discrimination by an algorithm, similar if not identical to the manner in which UNOS distributes anonymous deceased-donor organs under the current system.[7]

In this chapter we develop and evaluate a basic framework for the procurement and allocation of organs from compensated living providers. We then consider two different models of organ procurement and compensation. The first is a regulated, centralized system in which the federal government or a designated agency acts as the only authority with the power to provide financial compensation and allocate organs for transplantation.[8] The second approach is a regime in which the government issues a set of rules and regulations that provide a legal framework for private arrangements. Under this arrangement, the buyer and provider are free to set the value for their transaction.

In both cases, we discuss the effectiveness of the models in increasing the numbers of healthy kidneys used in transplantation, and how the models could be incorporated into the current system of organ procurement and allocation. We also discuss the role of physicians and transplant centers in the proper screening and selection of providers, post-transplant care, and other steps in the process of organ procurement. We do not enter into the many complex ethical issues involved in providing financial incentives for living organ providers, which are addressed in chapters 1, 5, and 6.

Basic Framework for a Compensation System

A number of common features must underlie any system of organ procurement; foremost among them are the safety of the providers, informed consent, and confidentiality of the transactions. The basic organizational features of the compensation models would rely heavily on the current system of deceased-donor allocation and recipient follow-up, as regulated by the Organ Procurement and Transplantation Network (OPTN) and administered by UNOS. Figure 3-1 presents an organizational chart of the basic framework. Each box in the diagram represents a different set of agents or agencies that would be involved in the procurement and transplantation of organs from compensated living providers. The evaluation, allocation, and follow-up of compensated providers would be the responsibility of the regionally based organ procurement organizations (OPOs). Currently, OPOs are linked to the centralized UNOS computer. They individually coordinate the logistics among the families of deceased donors, the organs that are procured, the transplant centers, and the potential transplant recipients within well-defined geographic areas.

In the proposed system, oversight of the OPOs' compensated-provider program would be conducted by a newly formed National Providers Registry (hereafter referred to as "the registry"), a centralized administrative agency set up under the auspices of the U.S. Department of Health and Human Services and separate from OPTN/UNOS. The current mechanism of oversight for procurement and distribution of deceased-donor organs would remain intact and operate in parallel. Kidney procurement from the provider, transplantation into the recipient, and medical follow-up for both

FIGURE 3-1

BASIC FRAMEWORK FOR COMPENSATED-PROVIDER PROGRAMS

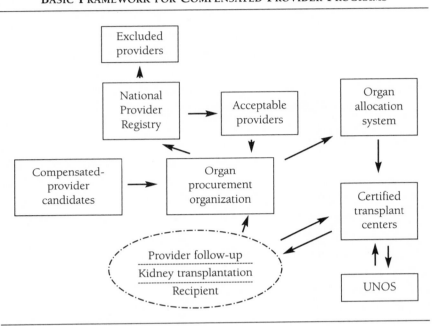

SOURCE: Authors' illustration.

would be the responsibility of the transplant center. In addition to overseeing the OPOs, the registry would maintain all data relevant to the compensated provider, including follow-up. Descriptions of the various agencies and their functions follow.

Organ Procurement Organizations. Currently, forty-eight OPOs accredited by the Association of Organ Procurement Organizations (AOPO) are located throughout the United States.[9] Assigning to the OPOs the responsibilities of provider screening, evaluation, and allocation in the new system would be in keeping with their current mission of:

> advocacy, support, and development of activities that will maximize the availability of organs and tissues and enhance the quality, effectiveness, and integrity of the donation process.[10]

OPOs presently manage and coordinate all aspects of deceased-donor organ procurement and allocation. Many are also involved in tissue procurement (skin, bone, heart valves, and so forth) from deceased donors. In addition, OPOs provide educational programs for hospitals, health-care personnel, and the general public in the area of organ and tissue donation and transplantation. These entities provide a critical interface between the deceased-donor organ and the transplant center and are highly regulated by a variety of state and federal agencies; for example, donor allocation within particular geographic areas follows the standard UNOS algorithm.[11] Consequently, OPOs have an intimate understanding of the donor allocation system and a close working relationship with the area transplant centers. They are uniquely positioned and qualified to expand their role to include evaluation and allocation of compensated providers.

Under our proposed system, the OPO would assume a primary role as liaison between the compensated-provider candidate and the transplant center, educating applicant providers about the transplantation process, risks of surgery, nature of recovery, and impact on future health, performing medical and psychological evaluations, and allocating providers based on the UNOS algorithm or other scheme devised by an independent body, such as the American Society of Transplant Surgeons. The OPO would be responsible for coordinating compensated-provider follow-up and for the reporting of immediate, short-term, and long-term follow-up health data to the National Provider Registry mentioned above. As in its present role in the allocation of deceased-donor organs, the OPO would be responsible as well for covering the costs associated with compensated-provider evaluation and allocation, charging the transplant center the costs incurred for allocation of the provider, and paying the provider once the organ is procured. In addition, the OPO would encourage compliance of the provider with intermediate and long-term health assessments by distributing payments as installments to be spread across the prescribed period of follow-up health checks.

To expand services to accommodate compensated providers, the OPO would contract with or hire health-care personnel, such as physicians, social workers, donor advocates, mental health experts, and others (as determined by national standards) to carry out the standardized evaluation of the compensated-provider candidate. Health-care providers employed by the OPO would serve the candidate organ provider, but have no authority over or, influence on the referral process to a particular listed candidate or transplant center. In this context, the current UNOS requirement for the provision of separate donor and recipient teams would easily be met. The healthcare providers, working under the direction of the OPO, would have only the compensated organ provider as their primary charge, as the potential recipient would be unidentified at this stage of the evaluation.

Compensated-provider evaluations would be performed at the OPO facilities (which might require modest expansion of current facilities). Most of the laboratory testing required is already performed by the OPO for deceased-donor evaluations, while radiological evaluation, cardiopulmonary testing, endoscopy services, and other specialty services outside of current OPO capability could be referred out on a consulting basis to any medical center or physician practice.

Transplant Centers. In any compensation model, the allocation of acceptable providers would only be made to existing transplant centers that had

- official registration as participating centers;

- Medicare certification for kidney transplantation;

- designation as members in good standing with OPTN/UNOS; and

- certification by UNOS in the performance of living-donor kidney transplantation.

A compensated kidney provider would be allocated to a listed transplant candidate based on current UNOS policy pertaining to deceased-donor organs. The transplant center at which the candidate is listed (allocation to candidates listed at multiple centers would default to the center with the longest wait time) would be provided with the comprehensive evaluation of the living provider conducted by the OPO; upon review the center would have the opportunity to accept or decline the compensated provider or request further testing. In cases where the center requested additional testing or declined the offer, the center would be required to submit written justification of its action to the OPO within a specified period of time. (For these situations, a formal process of review and action would need to be constructed.)

Upon acceptance of the allocation, the compensated provider would be interviewed, with final evaluation and scheduling taking place at the transplant center. Organ procurement and transplantation would then proceed in the traditional fashion. The transplant center would be responsible for postoperative care and treatment of any complications, either immediate or delayed, experienced by the provider.

National Provider Registry. The National Provider Registry, the proposed centralized administrative agency under the auspices of the U.S. Department of Health and Human Services and separate from OPTN/UNOS, would be charged with establishing and enforcing standardized criteria for evaluation, acceptance, and follow-up of compensated providers. Oversight would be provided by a panel constituted of health-care providers, legal representatives, kidney transplant recipients, public representatives, clergy, ethicists, and other compensated providers. Policy development would be accessible and transparent.

All compensated providers who presented themselves for evaluation and proceeded beyond the introductory phases (see below) would be registered in a database according to name, birth date, Social Security number, biological compatibility factors (such as blood type and tissue type, also known as HLA type),[13] and disposition of provider status (accepted, rejected, failed to complete evaluation, or declined to participate); and information necessary for the organ removal and transplant would be delivered to designated transplant centers. Follow-up health information and data on all compensated providers used for transplantation would be recorded. The registry would hold confidential all compensated-provider information according to current policy on patient confidentiality under the federal Health Insurance Portability and Accountability Act (HIPAA).[14]

Process of Compensated-Provider Evaluation, Allocation, and Follow-Up

Institution of a program of compensated providers would be well-publicized, with basic selection criteria announced and those interested in participating directed to any of the regionally based[15] OPOs for three phases of registration and assessment: the introductory phase, the data-acquisition phase, and the evaluation phase. Accepted providers would then be sent on to transplant centers for the allocation phase and completion of the transplant.

Introductory Phase. Protection of providers must be at the core of any proposed kidney transplantation network. Currently, living donors are evaluated by individual transplant centers using many different protocols and standards. This variability has recently prompted OPTN/UNOS to propose standard criteria for donor evaluation and acceptance, to which all transplant programs will be expected to adhere.[16]

In a market system, the fundamental task of ensuring adherence to such an established, transparent set of provider inclusion and exclusion criteria would still be performed by certified OPOs according to a standardized template for evaluation. Individuals interested in being providers would be referred to regional OPOs by any of the agents involved in the transplant network, by telephone, or through the Internet. They would be given an introductory overview, in print and multimedia formats, of the process of participating in the compensated-provider program, with a list of the tests to be performed and an outline of the sequential investigations and follow-up required. Those interested in pursuing evaluation would be required to receive, understand, and sign a consent form listing the requirements for participation, follow-up, data collection, and registration with the registry, as well as the risks associated with the evaluation and nephrectomy. A basic health questionnaire would then be completed.

Data Acquisition Phase. Having consented to all requirements, an individual who wished to proceed further with the process would be asked to register as a provider candidate by supplying primary-source documentation of his or her name, Social Security number, citizenship, address, and birth date, and to submit to testing for determination of blood and tissue (HLA) type. The identifying information would be used to track provider candidates throughout the process, becoming particularly important in preventing individuals rejected at one OPO from trying to gain access to the system at another. Further data collection would include candidate demographics, employment status, marital status, and medical and health history, among other items. This initial screening process would identify obvious contraindications or exclusion criteria for participation, such as diabetes or a history of high blood pressure.

Evaluation Phase. Compensated-provider candidates who completed the data acquisition phase without an obvious contraindication would be given appointments for comprehensive psychological, medical, and laboratory evaluations,[17] with the results assessed according to a standardized series of templates. Those accepted for participation would go on to receive the remaining invasive investigations, such as computed tomography (CT) angiogram, endoscopy, and cardiovascular testing, as indicated.

Upon completion of this last stage of the evaluation, compensated provider candidates would be reviewed by the medical review board at the OPO, whose assessment would, in turn, be presented to the registry oversight committee for final review. Acceptable candidates still interested in being providers would be educated in more detail about the process of nephrectomy and the risks and benefits of the surgical procedure, as well as the requirements for long-term follow-up, and the level and timeframe of compensation for their participation. A three-month cooling-off period would then give providers sufficient time to contemplate the risks involved, as well as the details of the surgery and recovery, and to provide an additional level of informed consent—or to drop out, if they should have second thoughts.

Allocation Phase. For provider candidates finally accepted into the program, organ distribution would be based, as previously indicated, on the current system used by UNOS for allocation of deceased-donor organs.[18] Because substantial immunological benefit and improved rates of patient and organ survival are associated with situations in which a total HLA match or a non-mismatch are found between a listed transplant candidate and an accepted compensated provider, they would be given high priority.

Once identified by the allocation algorithm, the provider candidate would be given the option of traveling to the transplant center at which the recipient was registered.[19] (A provider who declined because of the travel involved would be reassigned according to UNOS criteria for regional allocation of deceased-donor organs.) Upon identification of a recipient registered at an approved transplant center to which the provider was willing to go, that center would be notified of the provider's availability. The center would have to have been participating in the compensated-provider program, making its participation public, and complying with all regulations associated with the program. If these requirements were met, the provider's medical evaluation and testing data—all of which would have to comply with HIPAA regulations—would be forwarded to the transplant center, which would then decide whether to accept or decline the provider. If the center declined the provider, the reasons for the refusal would be placed on file with the registry. A provider who was refused for center-specific reasons, such as a weight or age limit, would be allocated to the next potential candidate in the queue at another participating center. This process would continue until the provider was accepted and the transplant accomplished.

Transplant Center. Upon acceptance by a transplant center of a compensated provider, the next step would be a meeting between the provider and the center's transplant team to discuss the risks and benefits of the surgical procedure, obtain consent for organ retrieval, and schedule the operation and transplant. Neither the candidate nor the transplant center would be obligated to continue the process if either or both parties had reservations. Withdrawal of participation and the justification for it would have to be communicated to the OPO, and all decisions not to proceed evaluated and recorded with the registry.

If the provider and the transplant center decided to proceed with the transplant, arrangements would be made according to the standard procedure for living-donor kidney transplantation. All activities between provider and recipient would be coordinated through third parties and the anonymity of both maintained. The compensated donor would be cared for by the transplant center until discharged from acute-care follow-up. At minimum, this would include the immediate care during the hospitalization associated with the nephrectomy and the outpatient postoperative care. If no complications resulted from the nephrectomy, the compensated provider would be discharged to continue routine follow-up through the OPO. If, however, complications were to occur (then or later), the transplant center would have to continue care until the provider had recovered.

Models of Financial Compensation in a Market System

Programs of compensation for living organ providers can take many forms and entail different degrees of regulation. As we have discussed, certain universal features are already in effect in the current system (for example, the role of the physician and transplant centers in the proper screening and selection of donors, post-transplant care, surgical techniques, and organ allocation and other steps of organ procurement). It is important to acknowledge, however, that different models have strengths and weaknesses that are modified by the socioeconomic, political, religious, and cultural aspects of different societies and, therefore, not applicable to all.

Here we consider a centralized system and a free-market operation as different versions of a market structure intended to increase the supply of transplantable organs.

Centralized System. The structure of a centralized market system would be analogous to that of the current organization for deceased-donor organs and would share all of the characteristics of the basic framework we have described above. The federal government would be the organizer, as Medicare and Medicaid expenditures for end-stage renal treatment already give it the largest financial investment in and potential savings from such a system. Moreover, much of the transplant organization is already regulated by government agencies at all levels.

A centralized arrangement would provide the most regulatory control over the institution of a new system of organ procurement, dictating the type and quantity of providers used, and all aspects of evaluation and allocation. All providers would receive the same fees and services, and all activities would be readily transparent. All participants would be afforded protection under the current legal system. A central body, the National Providers Registry, would be responsible for all components necessary to execute a kidney transplant from provider to recipient. Oversight function could be assumed by OPTN or a new agency that would interface with OPTN/UNOS.

Under such a system, many of the organizations currently operating for deceased-donor transplantation would be used and expanded. Potential providers would be evaluated by the current OPOs, as outlined above.

Criteria for participation would be prospectively defined and, depending on the stringency of the criteria regarding providers' age range (for example, between twenty-five and forty years), much of the testing normally required of older adults (such as mammograms, colonoscopies, or extended cardio-pulmonary evaluations) would be waived. Such high-threshold participation requirements should enable the organization to lower provider mortality risk, incidence of complications, and recovery time, in addition to extending the longevity of the transplanted kidney.

Certified transplant programs would be allowed to participate in the compensated-provider program. Provider allocation would follow the system currently in operation for deceased-donor organs. Consequently, all participating transplant programs would have equal access to an available provider. Anonymity between provider and recipient would be most feasible under a centralized system, as allocation of an organ would be made to a national or regional waiting list rather than being handled within an individual transplant center.

The OPOs would charge transplant programs a comprehensive fee for a provider kidney in much the same way they assign procurement charges (covering retrieval, preservation, transportation, and other acquisition costs) under the current system for deceased-donor kidneys. The fee for the compensated-provider transplant might be higher than for deceased donation because, in addition to the expense of expanding services for the program and provider evaluation, costs associated with provider candidates who did not end up providing organs would have to be amortized over the total number of providers and charged on a per-provider basis.

Provider compensation would be fixed in advance by the government (federal or state), which would serve as the single payer and prospectively determine the type and duration of payments.[20] The compensation could take any of a number of forms, including fixed payment or in-kind rewards, such as long-term health insurance, college tuition, or tax deductions, or a package that included some combination of these or other, equally valuable, alternatives.[21] Among other advantages, such in-kind rewards would almost surely be more politically palatable in the implementation of a new compensation program than offers of cash. The National Kidney Foundation (the dominant interest group in the transplantation field) is forcefully opposed to payment, and, given the failure of UNOS to support pilot investigations and the lack of outright endorsements from professional societies within the transplant field, there are no reputable entities to counter it.

The moral objections to compensating donors are discussed in depth elsewhere in this book,[22] but it is worth mentioning here that opposition to cash payment is commonly based on the worry that prospective donors will see it as an offer they cannot refuse and rush to surgery against their better judgment or true desire. The virtue of delayed, in-kind rewards is that they do not satisfy the economic needs of desperate people. Granted, most providers will be of lower-income status, but the combination of in-kind rewards instead of immediate cash—the form of remuneration that would appeal most to desperate individuals—with a months-long cooling-off period prior to surgery should neutralize concern about undue inducement.

For simplicity and transparency, however, a monetary payment would work best as the system developed. Monetary payments have proved to work well as compensation for sperm and egg providers, and they may prove to be a more effective motivator than in-kind rewards such as tax credits. A smoothly functioning pilot period of in-kind rewards might, however, allow the public to adjust to the very idea of compensation so that actual payment became more socially acceptable over time, especially if spread out over a number of years.

The registry would be in charge of setting a value for the monetary compensation. Building on the value-of-life literature, Becker and Elías have estimated that a $15,000 payment would be enough to attract a large pool of providers, while Matas and Schnitzler show that the public health system would break even with a $94,000 cost per provider.[23] Funding for direct payment or in-kind remuneration would be derived from the considerable savings accrued when patients exit the dialysis rolls.[24]

Several considerations are fundamental to all these schemes: the requirement for provider safety in the processes of evaluation, nephrectomy, and follow-up care, and for the safety of the recipient; justice and fairness in recipient access, organ allocation, and transplantation; protection under the law; and transparency of the entire process. A proposal for provider protections would have to guarantee long-term follow-up medical care, with the transplant center placed in charge of referring the provider to a medical center for further follow-up and required to report the referral to the registry and the OPOs. To ensure long-term follow-up, providers would receive 60 percent of their payment directly after the transplantation procedure, with the remaining 40 percent spread out over a period of five years, during which the registry and the OPOs would monitor their compliance with visits and observation. Small payments would be offered as incentives to providers to fill out questionnaires biannually for the next ten years, and for every five to ten years thereafter. Each provider would receive two-year term life insurance and disability insurance, as well as ongoing health care for medical matters related to transplantation.[25]

Free Market. An unregulated market for kidneys in the United States might be organized in several ways. One simple model is the private contract apparatus presently used by couples who seek women to serve as surrogate mothers. The prospective surrogate agrees to gestate a baby and then relinquish it to the couple, who become its adoptive parents. Although details about payment, prenatal care, and other matters are negotiated between the two parties and codified in a legal contract, the medical treatment is delivered by third parties (such as physicians and hospitals) that have their own practice codes and ethical guidelines.

In general, a legal free market in kidneys for transplantation would probably exhibit great flexibility in terms of the structure of the organizations that would act as intermediaries between transplant centers and providers. Certain features, however, would likely rely on the basic framework for the compensated-provider system already discussed. For instance, as information-sharing about potential providers resulted in important gains for both transplant centers and organ procurement agencies, a national registry of potential providers or an equivalent (perhaps decentralized) information-sharing system would likely emerge, bringing together all relevant information pertaining to potential and excluded providers.

In addition, minimum rules, such as those outlined within our basic framework, could be established to ensure that the roles of physicians and transplant centers in the proper screening and selection of donors, post-transplant care, and other steps of the process of organ procurement continued to be at the core of the system. For example, where a central agency might control organ procurement firms and establish some rules about their relationships with transplant centers, competition among these institutions in a completely decentralized system would likely ensure high standards in terms of compensated-providers' safety and post-transplant care.

In a free-market system, compensation for providers would be set at the levels that would eliminate the shortage of organs. As mentioned above, Becker and Elías have estimated such compensation at about $15,000. If government subsidies or private insurance covered payments to providers, a free market would encourage some patients to secure transplant organs legally rather than turning to the black market, particularly since the wait in the legitimate system would be sharply reduced.

It must be noted, however, that a traditional free-market approach generates ethical conundrums that a government-sponsored and financed compensation system averts; these are discussed at length elsewhere in this book. Pragmatically, we suspect that a free-market system is too controversial and will garner virtually no political support.

Conclusion

Since 1984, the formalized system of organ recovery and allocation in the United States has been dependent on a deficient model that has failed to procure the requisite number of kidneys for transplant. The continued reliance on an approach to organ acquisition that has been inadequate and outmoded for nearly a quarter of a century is medically unacceptable, morally indefensible, and financially unsound, especially when a reasonable solution exists in compensated providers.

In a system relying upon living donors or providers, the organs provided for transplantation would be of better quality and allocated on an elective basis, with a better possibility of close tissue-type matching. Under these conditions, transplant outcomes would be optimized because the transplantation of organs from the living is medically superior to deceased-donor transplantation.[26] Furthermore, transplants arranged in advance with living providers are more convenient, less costly, and less disruptive to the recipient and the transplant center than deceased-donor transplants, which are generally performed on an emergency basis upon the donor's sudden or unexpected death. A greater supply of organs for transplantation would decrease time spent on dialysis and improve patient- and organ-survival rates, as well as result in an overall savings in health-care expenditure for end-stage kidney disease services, even after adding the cost of the compensated donor.[27]

The present transplantation system imposes an intolerable burden on many very ill individuals who cannot afford to wait years until a suitable organ becomes available. A system for compensated living organ providers is the best available way to eliminate this wait and allow more such patients to survive.

Organ transplantation is the best form of therapy for end-stage kidney disease; organ donation from deceased donors is insufficient to meet the needs of people for transplantation; procurement of organs from living donors is already accepted and safe and ethically acceptable. The only issue left to resolve is how to ethically and socially facilitate a relationship between the suppliers of living organs and the candidates in need. In this chapter we have provided an operational outline of such a model.

4

Donor Compensation without Exploitation

James Stacey Taylor and Mary C. Simmerling

In March 2006, Eric De Leon of San Mateo, California, traveled to Shanghai, China, to get a new liver. The fifty-one-year-old construction supervisor was ineligible for a transplant in the United States because he had advanced hepatic cancer and was expected to live less than a year. Upon his return from the successful surgery, for which he'd raised the money in part by mortgaging the family home, the "transplant tourist" was stunned to find himself a reviled public figure, maligned in the *San Francisco Chronicle* as an "American Vampire," guilty of "moral depravity" for "us[ing] other people's parts."[1]

Sadly, this sort of outcry is understandable. A tragic fact of transplant tourism is that it often puts the "suppliers" of organs at considerable risk to their own well-being.[2] In India and the Philippines, for example, indigent citizens who sell their organs may be ill-informed, if not deceived, about the nature of the surgery, may receive no medical follow-up, and may be cheated out of promised payments.[3] In China, where Eric De Leon obtained his liver transplant, well-documented offenses are most egregious: organs are harvested from executed prisoners, some of them members of the Falun Gong, a persecuted spiritual sect.[4]

The overseas organ trade has been decried by the international medical community. The International Transplant Society, the World Health Assembly of the World Health Organization, and the World Medical Association all condemn commercial transactions in organs.[5] In 2004, the World Health Assembly resolved to make countries accountable for transplant activities by calling on member states to protect the most vulnerable from transplant tourism and the sale of tissues and organs.[6] More recently, in 2008, a meeting convened in Istanbul by the Transplantation Society and the International Society of Nephrology led to the *Declaration of Istanbul on Organ Trafficking and Transplant Tourism*, a document condemning policies or practices "in which an organ is treated as a commodity, including by being bought or sold or used for material gain."[7] Even in developed countries such as the United States, the prospect of compensating donors for their organs raises the specter of a society whose disadvantaged members feel unduly pressured by financial necessity to give up parts of their bodies to the advantaged who can afford them, while being unable to attain organs for transplantation when they themselves are in need.

Yet Eric De Leon was no worse than a desperately ill man who wanted to live long enough to see his young children grow up.[8] What should he have done? What should the multitudes of individuals in similar straits do to save their own lives? Most patients in need of organ transplants are suffering from renal failure. At least 200,000 are on waiting lists for kidneys worldwide, and many more have no access to transplantation or dialysis services at all. Without dialysis, patients cannot even survive long enough to be wait-listed.[9]

The remedy to the corrupt and unregulated system of exchange that poses such agonizing dilemmas to very sick people is its mirror image: a regulated and transparent regime that is backed by the rule of law and devoted to donor protection. Yet critics of proposals for such a system in the United States allege that a legal mechanism for compensating donors will only make the problems worse. The Transplantation Society issued an emphatic rejection of donor incentives:

> Organs and tissues should be freely given without commercial consideration or financial profit. . . . If the organ donation process were to be relegated to the laws of the market place, the less privileged might be exploited to improve the health of the more privileged, and the established safeguards surrounding altruistic donation would be compromised.[10]

Others have called a legalization regime a deceptive "Trojan horse" that conceals the same ethical transgressions plaguing the illicit market.[11] Still others have held that a system of compensated organ donation would lead to fewer, rather than more, transplant organs becoming available. They contend that the potential for enrichment would discourage people from donating altruistically and, in the end, the numbers of freely given organs lost would exceed those procured through the new compensation system.[12]

Predictions like these only muddy the donor organ debate and surely dampen enthusiasm for policy innovation among the public and politicians. In contrast, this chapter clarifies the considerable difference between a shadowy, unauthorized market and a regulated system of exchange. The allegation that a legalized market could stimulate a black market is the basis for strong ethical objection to experimentation with donor compensation. Thus, we begin by examining this proposition. Next, we turn to the specific failures of unregulated overseas markets in organs and assess the extent to which those consequences would be applicable to a regulated organ market in the United States. This consideration is relevant to another moral objection lodged against donor compensation: that a regulated system—simply because it would facilitate nonaltruistic transactions—would produce the same unacceptable outcomes as an unauthorized system. Finally, we conclude that the exploitative markets operating around the world are a manifestation of the widespread shortage of organs; they are not the inevitable outcome of lawful and regulated systems.

Will a Legal Market Lead to a Black Market?

Before examining the claim that a legal regime of donor compensation will spur illicit transactions, let us turn to vocabulary. The term "black market" refers to the trading of goods that are forbidden to be sold. India and Singapore, for example, both prohibit the selling and purchasing of organs, yet the practice continues within those countries in the form of an underground, illicit, or "black" market. By comparison, Pakistan does not have a law prohibiting the sale of organs.[13] There, the exchange of kidneys for cash occurs in a murky no man's land that is neither explicitly legal nor illegal. This transactional arena could be called an unregulated or unauthorized market. The situation in Pakistan shows that just because a country has no law *against* organ sales doesn't mean that it has laws necessary to actualize a safe and transparent system of exchange in which breaches of contract are enforceable.[14]

It is the undefined legal status of organ sales in various countries that makes it legally permissible for people like Eric De Leon to obtain transplants overseas. Agents or "transplant coordinators" in the United States and other countries—many of whom advertise on the Internet—deal with transplant hospitals in China, India, South Africa, Singapore, Pakistan, and South America.[15] A number of insurance companies in the United States offer "medical value travel" packages, which cover expenses and medical treatment overseas, plus sightseeing.[16] Fortunately for potential transplant tourists, physicians in America and elsewhere seem to have adopted a "won't endorse, can't condemn" policy. They rarely suggest the option to patients but are generally sympathetic to their plight and resume care when the patient returns.[17]

From the standpoint of the overseas donor, however, things are very different. Those considering selling a kidney rarely have personal physicians to advise them about the hazards of doing so and to care for them if they proceed.[18] In this harsh milieu, donors are at the mercy of lawless systems fraught with crime rings, corrupt middlemen and physicians, and hospital administrators willing to turn a blind eye to the source of the organs.[19] It is scenarios like these that have prompted critics to charge that a legal system of donor compensation could encourage exploitative and unjust organ markets both in the United States and developing countries.[20] "The acceptance of even a limited domestic organ market in the advanced nations," write two Indian physicians in a medical journal,

> will act as the proverbial thin end of the wedge and encourage adoption of commercial donation in the developing world. . . . Allowing such an activity in any corner of the world would open the doors for rampant exploitation of the underprivileged in areas that are already plagued by vast economic inequalities.[21]

This view was endorsed by the National Kidney Foundation in testimony before Congress in 2003. According to Francis L. Delmonico, testifying on behalf of the foundation, "A U.S. congressional endorsement for payment would propel other countries to sanction unethical and unjust standards."[22] Worse yet, opponents of legalizing compensation for transplant organs have argued, such legalization would stimulate black markets in human transplant organs, with all of their attendant injustices and ills.[23]

Such critiques are long on passion but short on critical analysis.[24] In particular, they never seem to explain how allowing compensation for transplant organs would lead to the ills they envisage, either at home or abroad. To fill this conceptual void, we must consider the circumstances under which a regulated regime in compensation could spur a commercial free-for-all, focusing in particular on the claim that it would stimulate illicit sales.[25]

We begin by identifying three objectives that would motivate a buyer to seek goods through an unauthorized market. First, a buyer might need to purchase something that is not available through legal means or whose supply is rationed under tight control. Second, a buyer might want to conceal evidence of a purchase (in the case, for example, of an individual who obtains painkillers or Viagra online, or a gun purchaser who doesn't want to register the gun with the police). Third, a buyer might seek the item at a cheaper price.[26]

How do these circumstances relate to compensated donation? The obvious seduction of the overseas trade is the promise of a scarce good. The other objectives, however, do not apply. The desire to make a purchase secretively, for example, can almost surely be ruled out. Undergoing renal transplantation is not a shameful activity. Nor are there any cost savings to be had if the state or federal government, not the patient, is the purchaser.[27] Moreover, the government would set the prices in a well-regulated system, so there would be no point in trying to obtain organs from illicit sources. Donors and recipients alike would surely prefer a system that protects them from force or fraud, especially when technical error can truly be a matter of life or death.[28] Indeed, legalizing markets in human organs would most likely reduce, rather than increase, such trafficking-related abuses by providing a person who might currently be tempted to buy a kidney in a black market with a legal (and safer) way to obtain one.[29]

Granted, there is a small subset of individuals who might find unauthorized channels attractive even if a safe and legal compensation system were in effect. These are people who have no means to pay for a transplant, perhaps because they cannot afford private health insurance, are not eligible for coverage by Medicare or Medicaid, or are not otherwise able to secure access to government-provided health care. These individuals are unfortunate, indeed; but the chances of their purchasing kidneys from unauthorized markets are slim, as the costs associated with organ purchase, implantation surgery, and immunosuppressant medication would simply be beyond their reach. Thus, legalizing a market in kidneys is not likely to stimulate a black market, because the only people who would be motivated to buy in one probably could not afford to do so.

Objections to Donor Compensation

Black market failures are vividly illustrated by the case of organ sales in India. Madhav Goyal of the Johns Hopkins School of Public Health and his research team conducted a detailed evaluation of donor outcomes in that country.[30] Their 2002 study of kidney sellers in Chennai, published in the *Journal of the American Medical Association*, is frequently cited as evidence that paid donors are highly vulnerable to exploitation.[31]

India banned sales of organs in 1994 to curtail the organ trade and limit donors to blood relatives and others who had been specifically approved. But because the law permitted unrelated individuals to donate if they signed a form saying they had not received money, brokers merely began encouraging prospective donors to claim they were not being paid.[32] By the time of their study, Goyal and colleagues found, corrupt brokers had become commonplace, with donors sometimes receiving only a portion of the money promised them. According to some reports, moneylenders would insist that debtors sell kidneys to pay off their debts. Moreover, they could threaten to withhold additional credit from those who still had two kidneys. The research team suggested that poor people did not, in fact, overcome poverty as a result of the sale of their kidneys. Many donors reported a worsening in their economic status after donation, with the annual family income declining by one-third—this despite an improvement in the overall economic status of others in their communities during the same time period. Moreover, even though 91 percent of interviewed donors sold kidneys to pay off debts, three-fourths were still in debt within six years of organ removal. About one in nine donors reported a decline in health.[33]

These hazardous aspects of organ trafficking underscore the most fundamental ethical condition of living-organ transplantation: that individuals who give organs—for enrichment or not—should be no worse off after giving than they were before. "A story about kidney sales in India may sound distant in many other parts of the world," says Jeffrey Kahn of the Center for Bioethics, University of Minnesota, "but proposals to test limited markets for kidneys in the U.S. mean that these lessons deserve a hard look."[34] Based upon their knowledge of problems that occur in illicit markets, opponents worry that in a donor compensation system, individuals will be coerced into donating organs; that they will be unable to give informed consent for donating their organs; that they will misrepresent their eligibility to donate; that the poor will supply the rich with organs; that donors will be worse off financially than they were before; that the quality of medical conditions will be unreliable for paid donors; and that fewer organs for transplantation will be secured than before the system was instituted. Let us examine these fears one by one, and show how a legitimate compensation system would neutralize them.

Individuals Will Be Coerced into Donating Organs. Some claim that the decision to sell organs would not be free in a donor compensation system because the introduction of financial inducements fundamentally changes the motivations of donors. They act out of a need for money rather than out of moral duty or compassion. "A poor person feels compelled to risk death for the sole purpose of obtaining monetary payment for a body part," write Francis L. Delmonico and colleagues.[35]

Are prospective donors who are impoverished or living in near-poverty coerced into giving up their organs by the lure of compensation? Before engaging this important question—perhaps the most pressing of all objections to rewarding donors—let us define coercion. In its classic form, coercion is a gun to one's head; it involves a physical threat to an individual (for example, hand over your money or be killed) or the threat of a bad outcome for refusing to comply (for example, do this or else lose your job).[36] Yet a person who refuses to give a kidney for payment is not diminished or harmed in any fashion. His circumstances may be dire to begin with, but he is no worse off if he holds on to his kidney.

A more precise term to describe the nature of the offer of reward for an organ is "undue inducement." As compared to a reasonable inducement (for example, a big discount sale at an expensive store in which one would not normally shop), an undue inducement is an excessive offer of reward for taking an action (for example, having an organ removed) that one would otherwise object to doing. Individuals may act contrary to their own desires, violate their own personal values, or knowingly undertake a risk that is considerable.[37] Because the offer is so compelling, it alters their ability to exercise proper judgment and thereby threatens informed consent, especially if they cannot assess the risk appropriately.

Yet the fact that potential donors are motivated by financial gain rather than by altruism is not sufficient to show they are acting less than fully voluntarily, that their autonomy is impaired through pressure applied to their will, or that they are being exploited.[38] Indeed, perhaps it is exploitative not to compensate donors. As altruistic kidney donor Virginia Postrel has written,

> Expecting people to take risks and give up something of value without compensation strikes me as a far worse form of exploitation than paying them. I don't expect soldiers or police officers to work for free, and I don't think we should base our entire organ donation system on the idea that everyone but the donor should get paid. Like all price controls, that creates a shortage—in this case, a deadly one. And while giving up a kidney has risks, it is no more risky and far less emotionally fraught than being a surrogate mother.[39]

Furthermore, a compensation program can circumvent the risk of undue inducement by not catering to the desperate. Such individuals desire cash and want it immediately. The proposed system would establish a months-long period of medical screening and education. It would also provide in-kind rewards, or cash paid out in modest amounts over a long period of time (a strategy which, incidentally, would also ensure that donors return for follow-up care). Such a system of compensation would probably not be attractive to people who might otherwise rush to flawed judgment—and surgery—on the promise of a large sum of instant cash.

Thus, a legal system of compensation with strict donor protections creates conditions in which the decision to relinquish a kidney can be informed and influenced by an offer rather than distorted by it.

Donors Will Not Give Informed Consent. Overseas brokers and hospitals have, indeed, exploited poorly educated individuals who were ignorant of the medical procedures involved in organ donation. Although such prospective donors might have signed consent forms, it is hard to imagine that many did so in a fully informed manner. By contrast, a regulated system of donor compensation would involve detailed education of prospective donors about the procedures involved and the risks they would be assuming.[40]

Individuals Will Misrepresent Their Eligibility to Donate. The National Kidney Foundation and others have expressed the concern that people will lie about their health status to be allowed to donate for compensation, thus posing a threat to recipients of possibly diseased organs.[41] This is, indeed, a legitimate warning in the context of unregulated markets where organ recipients have no legal recourse against unscrupulous organ donors or organ brokers, but it is inapplicable to a regulated system of compensation for organ donation for three reasons. First, it is based on the image of desperate third-world donors who are willing to put themselves at risk for cash. A regulated system of compensation would be structured so that the incentives offered would not appeal to the economically desperate—in short, there would be no lump-sum cash payments—and so they would not appeal to the persons with the most motivation to lie. Second, even if prospective donors were motivated to lie about their medical histories, they would be required to undergo rigorous testing over a period of several months to ensure they had no communicable diseases and that their organs were suitable for transplantation. Third, transplant centers could require prospective donors to provide them with the most recent five years of their medical records and permission to consult with their current physicians. Finally, both organ donors and health-care professionals could be made legally liable (both criminally and civilly) for any harm incurred by a patient as a result of receiving a diseased or substandard organ. This would provide a powerful incentive for all who are directly involved in the procurement of organs to ensure their quality.[42]

The Poor Will Supply the Rich. According to anthropologist Nancy Scheper-Hughes, who tracks the global trade in human organs, overseas organ markets are a glaring example of "medical apartheid" between organ givers and receivers.[43] "In general," she writes, "the movement and flow of living donor organs—mostly kidneys—is from South to North, from poor to rich, from black and brown to white, and from female to male bodies."[44] Characterizing the nature of this breach of social justice, a *Washington Post* journalist declares that "compensation for organs might exacerbate the differences [between rich and poor], turning the poor into surgical ward slaves or feudal donors for the rich."[45]

These descriptions do bear some weight. Yet a government-regulated system in which organs are allocated according to the current criteria of the United Network for Organ Sharing (UNOS) would ensure that all recipients benefit according to standard guidelines. Indeed, the economic demographic of candidates awaiting kidneys in the United States might not be radically discrepant from the status of the average donor.[46] As such, then, a regulated system of donor compensation would be neither racist nor classist in the ways that Scheper-Hughes implies. This is because, first, both donor and recipient would be given equal access to health care; and, second, in such a regulated system, all potential recipients would be favored equally. The donor compensation proposal would contain provisions for binding legal contracts. There would be no role for independent brokers.

Furthermore, such a regulated system would establish a uniform protocol for donor evaluation and post-transplant follow-up of compensated donors. In the current system, each institution applies its own selection criteria for the donor, and there is often little to no medical surveillance of the donor. Yet even with good follow-up, the donor has little incentive to make post-donation visits to the doctor beyond the immediate aftermath of the surgery. Contractual obligations of donor and institution would result in required patient follow-up and implementation of standard post-donation tests by each hospital. With respect to the well-being of donors, then, the model of compensated donation that is developed here would be superior to the current altruistic system.

Donors Will Be Worse Off Financially. Participants in the organ trade are often desperately poor, living on the edge of financial ruin. As Goyal demonstrated, they are also often worse off after kidney removal than before, for several reasons. First, the operation itself can pose obstacles to long-term gain. Surgeons in third-world countries commonly use a so-called retroperitoneal flank approach to remove the kidney—a primitive surgical technique that involves a nine-inch incision running from the top of the hip to the base of the ribs. The difference in the rate of healing compared to donors in developed countries who undergo a minimally invasive laparoscopic procedure is significant. Furthermore, most donors are laborers. It may be several weeks before a patient with a nephrectomy can return to work. When heavy manual labor is involved, the delay is even longer. With no money being earned during recuperation, no guarantee that medical complications will receive attention, and no assurance that jobs will be held for them (conditions which, for example, characterize Iran's legal system of donor compensation), it is no surprise that donors rarely enjoy financial benefit.[47]

This outcome, sad as it is, has little relevance to the donor compensation model proposed here. First, compensated U.S. donors would undergo a much less invasive procedure. Second, care of surgical and medical complications would be ensured. Third, expenses, including lost wages, would be covered.

The Quality of Medical Conditions Will Be Unreliable. The short-term medical status of patients who receive transplants abroad varies, depending upon the quality of the physicians and health-care facilities. A small sample of U.S. patients who have traveled overseas presents a high rate of post-transplant infections; reports on recipients from other countries are even less encouraging, with significant rates of mortality and infection with HIV and hepatitis B.[48] By comparison, within a legal and regulated environment, compensated donors and recipients would receive care in the same facilities and performed according to the same standards as those accorded to traditional altruistic donors. Presumably, in the United States, programs to perform living-donor kidney transplantation require extensive medical and psychological evaluations of potential donors to determine their medical suitability. A compensatory system would do the same and also build in medical follow-up for the uninsured donor, a clear advantage over the status quo.

Fewer Organs for Transplantation Will Be Secured. While it is possible that a system of paid compensation would reduce the number of kidneys given for free, this does not mean that altruistic donation would dry up. As philosopher Mark J. Cherry notes, many of "the motivations supporting such donations are likely to maintain the same force regardless of the existence of a for-profit market: love, beneficence, loyalty, gratitude, guilt, or avoidance of the shame of failing to donate."[49]

Moreover, a considerable body of evidence shows that even if altruistic donation were to decrease, the number of organs procured for transplant would not suffer an overall decline. A case in point is the system of compensating unrelated kidney donors that was introduced in Iran in 1988. In this system, potential kidney recipients who can find no biologically related donors are referred to the Dialysis and Transplant Patients Association (DATPA). If the patient does not receive a deceased-donor kidney within six months, DAPTA identifies a compatible live, unrelated, compensated kidney donor.[50] The donor is then compensated for the organ with a fixed amount (around $1,200), paid by the state. The donor also receives a year's worth of health insurance to cover conditions related to the surgery, as well as a payment from the organ recipient himself of around $2,300–$4,500; the precise amount is determined beforehand through the association.[51]

How did the Iranian system affect altruistic donation? It did, indeed, lead to a decline in the number of transplant kidneys given by biological relatives.[52] But the volume of kidneys procured from compensated donors more than made up for this reduction. Indeed, by 1999, Iran appeared to have eliminated its transplant waiting list.[53] Notably, the opposite dynamic was observed in India: After the country banned organ sales in 1994, several hospitals in Tamil Nadu reported a decline in the number of kidney transplants they were able to perform.[54]

Conclusion

It goes without saying that illicit overseas markets in human organs are often morally reprehensible. But their worst features hold little relevance for the development of a regulated and tightly supervised program in the United States. Indeed, the dangerous commercial organ markets operating around the world are manifestations of the widespread organ shortage, not the products of lawful and regulated systems. Yet without legitimate means of expanding the donor pool, trafficking will proceed apace—a prospect harmful not only to donors but also to the despairing patients who are reluctant participants in a corrupt enterprise.

Despite the florid rhetoric about regulated markets spawning a rapacious commercial trade that will run roughshod over the health and safety of desperate and unwitting donors, the commonsense arguments in favor of compensation and the available empirical evidence all pose a serious conceptual challenge to alarmist forecasts. If anything, the depredations of the underground market attest to the need for testing a legal mode of donor compensation. Whatever risks did remain would still be overwhelmed by the volume and enormity of abuses that occur in the current underground market. Inaction will only perpetuate these abuses. "Tragedy becomes complicity," writes nephrologist Benjamin Hippen, "when one fully understands that the public policy failures in organ procurement of the developed countries provide a robust economic foundation of organ trafficking in the developing world."[55]

5

Concerns about Human Dignity and Commodification

Sally Satel

In early 2006, Matt Thompson of San Jose, California, decided to give a kidney to Sonny Davis, a sixty-five–year-old physicist living in Menlo Park. Thompson was moved to donate after reading an impassioned plea from Davis's wife, who had sent 140 letters to friends and relatives asking them to consider helping her husband. One of the recipients happened to be a colleague of Thompson's who passed it along, thinking he just might heed the call.[1] Sure enough, Thompson, a devout young Christian and former missionary, contacted the transplant program to volunteer.

But the transplant program at Kaiser Permanente of Northern California turned him down. It would not allow Thompson to undertake the risk of surgery for the sake of a stranger. Had Davis been a family member or a good friend, he would have been acceptable to the program. Thompson was frustrated and surprised, but he and Davis were determined. According to the *San Jose Mercury News*, they "knew they had to forge a bond that would assure Davis' surgeons that Thompson was donating his kidney for the right reasons."[2] This meant, among other things, proving that Thompson would not profit financially. So the two developed a relationship and convinced the transplant program that no money was secretly being exchanged. On November 14, 2006, the transplant finally took place.

Far more than a human interest tale of a stranger opening his heart to a suffering soul, the story of Sonny Davis and Matt Thompson draws back the curtain on the culture of the organ transplant establishment. In fine detail, we see how transplant professionals would have allowed a sixty-five-year-old man to languish on dialysis for years or die—a strong probability given his age—while waiting for a kidney, out of fear that he might be remunerating someone for an act that would save his life. And what happened at the University of California at San Francisco (where Davis was transferred after the Kaiser program abruptly closed)[3] was not an isolated example, as may be surmised from the title of a 2007 *Wall Street Journal* article: "Why It's Hard to Give Away a Kidney: Most Hospitals Avoid Donors Who Want to Help Strangers, Wary of Motives and Fearing that the Neediest Aren't Served."[4]

While there is no evidence that Sonny Davis ever tried to purchase a kidney, surely others have contemplated doing so, and the pressing question remains: Is it morally justifiable to threaten a critically ill person with prison, let alone death, for simply enriching a donor?[5] The answer, according to some, is that exchanging an organ for anything of material value is an affront to human dignity, and that this is an immoral act.

This chapter delves into the deeply held convictions underlying the contention that donor compensation is intrinsically wrong—even if good comes from it, even if no one is exploited. It considers the concept of human dignity and the meaning of commodification and challenges the belief that human worth is inevitably corroded under a regime of compensation.

I conclude that transplant professionals sabotage their own cause—to alleviate suffering and save lives—when they extol altruism as the only acceptable motive for donation, and when they promote a particular ideal of human dignity as the only permissible guide to policy.

Dying for Dignity

In 2002, a group of physicians and bioethicists writing in the *New England Journal of Medicine* rejected the idea of material incentives for organ donation. "We do not endorse as public policy the sale of the human body through prostitution of any sort, despite the purported benefits of such a sale [of an organ] for both the buyer and the seller," they declared.[6] The lead author of the *Journal* article was transplant surgeon Dr. Francis Delmonico. The following year Delmonico represented the National Kidney Foundation, the major renal disease group in the United States, at a hearing before a U.S.

House of Representatives subcommittee. Under consideration was proposed legislation that would have allowed pilot studies of incentives. Delmonico told the committee that

> any attempt to assign a monetary value to the human body or its body parts, even in the hope of increasing organ supply, diminishes human dignity and devaluates the very human life we seek to save. . . . The NKF believes that it is impossible to separate the ethical debate of financial incentives for non-living donation from the unethical practice of selling human organs.[7]

This statement echoes the sentiments of bioethicist Cynthia Cohen, who declares that rewarding donors "denies embodied human dignity . . . and would violate a fundamental conviction at the core of our life together: that we should not treat human beings and integral aspects of their bodies as commodities."[8] Thus, exchanging a kidney for something of value violates the dignity of all involved—the donor who treats his body as a collection of spare parts (and himself as a means to an end), the society that permits him to do so, and the recipient who benefits from the dire economic circumstances of another.

The concept of human dignity pervades the controversy surrounding donor compensation. Though its significance may seem self-evident, "human dignity" is not sharply defined and is sometimes downright slippery. In the spring of 2008, for instance, Harvard psychologist Steven Pinker penned a sharp critique entitled "The Stupidity of Dignity." The title is a play on the name of a 1997 essay—"The Wisdom of Repugnance"—written by Leon Kass, the former chairman of the President's Council on Bioethics, and published in *The New Republic*.[9] Kass coined the term "wisdom of repugnance" to refer to the notion that deep reactions of disgust to an idea or practice (stem cell cloning was the particular subject of his essay) should be interpreted as evidence of its intrinsically harmful nature.

The impetus for Pinker's long and bristling essay, also published in *The New Republic*, was a recent report of the President's Council called *Human Dignity and Bioethics*. "The problem," according to Pinker, "is that 'dignity' is a squishy, subjective notion, hardly up to the heavyweight moral demands assigned to it."[10] He notes that he is not the first to challenge the coherence of the concept. In 2003 bioethicist Ruth Macklin, whom Pinker describes as "fed up with loose talk about dignity" by the President's Council, wrote an editorial in the *British Medical Journal* called "Human Dignity is a Useless Concept."[11] Macklin, he says, argued that bioethics had done just fine with the interrelated principles of personal autonomy, human rights, and respect for persons.

"The concept of dignity is a mess," Pinker claims bluntly. He identifies several features of dignity which, he says, should disqualify it as a foundational principle for bioethics. He points out, for example, that our definition of dignity is unstable, changing with social norms both within and across cultures. This kind of variability makes it a poor touchstone.

Consider that the meaning of dignity in the context of commerce varies over time. In his essay, "What Money Can't Buy: The Moral Limits of Markets," political philosopher Michael Sandel writes about "the extension of markets and of market-oriented thinking into spheres of life once thought to lie beyond their reach."[12] He cites as examples the privatization of prisons and the commercialization of hospitals, governments, and universities.

Many practices that now involve valuation were once considered immoral, repugnant, or undignified.[13] Until well into the thirteenth century, for example, the Catholic Church considered it a sin to charge interest on loans. Throughout much of the history of modern Europe—as, indeed, in ancient Greece—there was a common aristocratic prejudice against earning wages, as legal scholar Martha Nussbaum notes. And up until the early nineteenth century, it was considered inappropriate to pay female performing artists.[14] Adam Smith referred specifically to "players, opera-singers, opera-dancers," when he wrote in 1776 of "some very agreeable and beautiful talents of which the possession commands a certain sort of admiration; but of which the exercise for the sake of gain is considered, whether from reason or prejudice, as a sort of public prostitution."[15] Yet today, Nussbaum writes, "few professions are more honored than that of opera singer. . . . Nor do we see the slightest reason to suppose that the unpaid artist is a purer and truer artist than the paid artist."[16]

Another example of changing views of valuation concerns the pricing of life itself. Social economist Viviana Zelizer describes how early life insurance was seen as the merchandising of life. The concept was introduced in the eighteenth century but did not gain momentum until around 1840, when it found acceptance as a way to aid widows and orphans; the industry grew swiftly after that point.[17] The discomfort with selling organs is curious insofar as the practice of assigning values to body parts is ancient. The Code of Hammurabi provides an elaborate schedule of compensation for them; for example, it specifies that if an individual should "knock out the teeth of a freed man, he shall pay one-third of a gold mina."[18]

Ultimately, Pinker argues that dignity only proves useful as a moral guide if it is understood in the very specific sense of avoiding unnecessary humiliation and treating others with respect. But within that narrow context, the concept becomes "a mundane matter not a contentious moral conundrum." Basically, dignity "amounts to treating people in the way that they wish to be treated"—an application of the principles of autonomy and reciprocity (that is, doing unto others).[19] It boils down to no more than an unassailable imperative to treat people humanely—to regard them as an end, not a means.

In a 2002 article in *Transplantation*, the American Society of Transplant Surgeons states that incentives for living donors would "unacceptably commercialize the value of human life by commodifying donated organs."[20] Cited in the article are the sentiments of Pope John Paul II, who told the International Congress of the Transplantation Society that "any procedure which tends to commercialize human organs or to consider them as items of exchange or trade must be considered morally unacceptable, because to use the body as an 'object' is to violate the dignity of the human person."[21]

A close look at the pontiff's language is revealing, specifically the conditional phrase, "to use the body as an 'object.'" He appears to be saying that dignity is conditional upon how we regard the donor. Arguably, this perspective actually weighs against the view that compensating people for their organs is wrong; for if dignity can be eroded by *using* donors *as* objects, then, conversely, dignity can be preserved by doing the opposite—that is, by thinking of donors as lifesavers, by scrupulously protecting their safety, and by treating them with gratitude for their acts and with respect for their capacity to make considered judgments about their own best interests.

This humane approach contrasts with what British philosopher Stephen Wilkinson calls the "commodifying attitude"—a disposition that regards commercial exchanges as sterile and uncaring, denying the thoughts and feelings of the provider of a thing and relating to that thing solely in terms of its instrumentality and interchangeability (in the sense of one widget being as good as the next).[22] Legal scholar Margaret Radin proposes the notion of "incomplete commodification," in which some contested things, such as organs, can be bought and sold, but only under carefully regulated circumstances.[23] This complements Wilkinson's claim that the context in which something is sold can affect our perception of it.

What's more, compensation can even *promote* dignity. An individual who acts to enhance the well-being of another demonstrates an awareness of the other's value and uniqueness. That awareness also says something about that individual, that he or she is the sort of person who is capable of appreciating the humanity of another and responding to it. In the Kantian tradition, that appreciative capacity reflects moral agency, and moral agents have dignity and worth.[24] Or, expressed in less technical terms, that person is a "mensch." Of course, one reason we admire firefighters, salaried though they are, is that they put themselves at some inconvenience or even grave risk for the sake of others. The same extends to the compensated kidney donor.

Thus, there is nothing mystical or transcendent about the manifestation of dignity within the context of donor compensation. We can address justifiable anxieties about a commercial exchange involving humans and their alienable organs by conducting those transactions under the strictest conditions of decency and accountability. Indeed, the very defense of a regulated market in kidneys depends on nothing less than the respectful treatment of donors as beings capable of making thoughtful decisions about their bodies in order to serve their own—and others'—best interests.

Does Money Taint?

In "What Money Can't Buy," Michael Sandel calls rationales such as those in opposition to organ compensation "arguments from corruption"—objections that proceed from the belief that "certain moral and civic goods are diminished or corrupted if bought and sold for money."[25] Is assigning a monetary value to an organ some kind of affront to notions of human worth? "An organ is priceless, and payment for any organ would be so incommensurate to its worth to the recipient that it would somehow cheapen it," physician and bioethicist Jay Baruch of Brown University writes.[26] What Baruch and others fail to take into account, however, is that we routinely assign valuation to the body. Human blood plasma is collected primarily though paid donation. A person who serves as an egg or sperm donor gets paid for giving gametes and a surrogate mother for carrying someone else's child. Personal injury lawyers seek damages for bodily harm to their clients. The Veterans Administration puts a price on physical disabilities. We pay for justice in the context of personal injury litigation in the form of legal costs, and for our very lives in the form of medical fees. There is little reason to believe—nor tangible evidence to suggest—that these practices depreciate human worth or undermine human dignity in any way.

In fact, the reverse can happen. Failure to pay for something, the *very opposite* of offering money, can engender moral outrage. Consider how angry and demoralized injured plaintiffs and combat veterans become when their claims for disability payments are denied. It is *because* they value their bodies and their functions so dearly that they demand restitution for harm. Similarly, when an insurance company refuses to pay for liver or heart transplant surgery, it is saying, in effect, that the patient's very life is not worth the money the treatment would cost.

Critics of donor compensation worry, in addition, that the promise of a reward will induce people to give organs for the wrong reasons. "Avoidance of self-interest on behalf of the donor must be implicit" in the screening process, a position paper of the National Kidney Foundation declared in 1991. A decade and a half later, not much has changed. In 2006, the Institute of Medicine acknowledged that "altruism—a motivation for action that is concerned only about others' welfare—is sometimes viewed as the predominant and only acceptable motivation for donation in the current system."[27]

In reality, though, mixed motives are as likely to accompany "gifts" as they are to characterize paid acts—as, for example, in the case of a relative who gives a kidney out of guilt.[28] Guilt may not be the ideal motivation for the gift—but it does not lessen the value of the organ to the recipient, and neither would compensation. When a woman sells her eggs to an infertility clinic or receives money for carrying someone else's child in her womb, she helps to fulfill her clients' dearly held wish for parenthood. This phenomenon of giving motivated by a mix of altruism and a desire for compensation is nicely captured in an ad seen in a subway station: "Be a Sperm Donor. Good Cause/Good Money. Help an Infertile Couple."[29] Similarly, many women are attracted to paid surrogacy because they love motherhood and sympathize with women for whom it does not come easily. According to Sandra Hodgson, a family law attorney and director of Northwest Surrogacy Center in Portland, Oregon, compensation is a draw, but not the only one. "Money is never the sole factor," she told a reporter.[30] A study on Iranian kidney donors who received payment (Iran is the only country that authorizes organ sales) found that many donors expressed marked distress over a perceived lack of gratitude from the patients who received their kidneys.[31] Their desire for recognition is compelling evidence that these "sellers" saw the transaction as being worth more than the price placed on the kidneys themselves.

To suggest that financial and humanitarian motives reside in discrete realms is unrealistic—whether one performs a task for material benefit or performs it for free, mixed motives such as the above are often involved. Moreover, it is unclear how their commingling is inherently harmful. The goodness of an act is not diminished because someone was paid to perform it. Examples in support of this point abound: The great teachers who enlighten us and the doctors who heal us inspire no less gratitude because they are paid. A salaried firefighter who risks his or her life to save a child trapped in a burning building is no less heroic than a volunteer firefighter. Soldiers accept military pay while pursuing a patriotic desire to serve their country. The desire to do well by others while enriching oneself at the same time is as old as humankind. Indeed, the very fact that generosity and remuneration so often intertwine can be leveraged to good ends: to increase the pool of transplantable organs, for instance.

And what about the "good" itself? Doesn't its value transcend its price tag? Consider the example of a woman who owns a Picasso. She considers it priceless yet has it insured, a process requiring an appraisal of its monetary value. If the painting is destroyed, she will be compensated, but she will never be fully repaid for the loss, because the artwork holds vast personal meaning. Lori Andrews of Chicago-Kent College of Law offers another compelling illustration:

> Even though it would have been possible for me to have paid $10,000 for a surrogate mother to gestate my son and $4 an hour to a babysitter to care for him, I [would still] clearly think of my relationship with him as special and not having a market value.[32]

Clearly, something can have a price but still be invaluable. This is because commercial transactions are embedded in social contexts which endow acts of exchange, as well as the very goods that are being exchanged (a Picasso, a baby, an organ), with great moral significance.

Returning for a moment to donor motivation, it is true that not every blood plasma, egg, or sperm donor cares about the well-being of the recipient. Even if payment is offered as a symbol of gratitude, the donor may engage in the transaction simply as a way to make money. But why should that matter? When the Internal Revenue Service offers tax deductions for charitable contributions, the charity that receives the money is essentially uninterested in the donor's motivations. Whether it is a heartfelt contribution or one made simply for the tax break, the charity is happy to cash the check, knowing how much good the money will do for the needy. That is its primary, if not exclusive, concern. The same principle should apply to compensated organ donation. With the safety and freedom of the donor protected, the relevant emphasis should be on increasing the supply of donated kidneys to reduce suffering and save lives.[33]

And what about Michael Sandel's distinction between things that can't be bought and things that *shouldn't* be bought? I believe the moral limits of markets are reached when the good in demand—the kidney, in this case—is rendered dysfunctional by the very act of paying the provider for it. That is why it is impossible to "buy" someone's friendship, love, or passion—none of them "functions" properly unless given freely. Nor can one buy a Nobel Prize, because it will lose its meaning as an honor. "Market exchange immediately dissolves the good that you are seeking," as Sandel puts it.[34] But a kidney is different. Once transplanted, it performs its essential functions of filtering waste from the blood and maintaining water and electrolyte balance, whether it is paid for or not. Indeed, not only does the kidney retain its function (which is obvious), but the humanity of both donor and recipient is retained—perhaps even enhanced—whether it is paid for or not.

Sandel agrees that money *can* buy a kidney, and that the good survives the selling, but then goes on to ask whether it should be allowed to. "Does money degrade or corrupt the good at stake?" he asks. He asks whether we should allow the selling of votes or military duty and concludes that doing so would corrupt the ideals of citizenship and civic virtue. On buying kidneys, though, Sandel is, in the end, inscrutably silent. If there is a sacred principle threatened by rewarding a donor who is protected and informed and whose actions save a life, he does not offer one.

Romanticizing Altruism

The debate surrounding incentives for organ donation sometimes resembles a titanic struggle between uplift and greed. "As a rule, the debate is cast as one in which existing relations of selfless, altruistic exchange are threatened with replacement by market-based, for-profit alternatives," observes Kieran Healy, a sociologist at the University of Arizona.[35] The National Kidney Foundation, we have seen, warns against "self-interest on behalf of the donor."[36] The ethics committee of the American Society of Transplantation perpetuates an either/or approach to the issue: "Altruism should not be abandoned for an organ system that would commodify human organs."[37] Thomas A. Shannon, a professor of religion and social ethics, writes, "I would think it a tragedy if . . . we tried to solve the problem of the organ shortage by commodification rather than by the kindness of strangers who meet in the community and recognize and meet the needs of others in generosity."[38]

As we have already observed, however, the motives behind the acts both of giving and selling are often mixed, and philosopher James Childress rejects these as false choices. "Just as the economic model of human motivation is deficient," he writes, "so is the model that sees only unadulterated altruism in the donation of organs. A more realistic conception of human motivations, sentiments, symbols, and actions . . . should guide all public policies in this area."[39]

To be sure, unadulterated altruism is real. In the interest of full disclosure, I must mention that I became a beneficiary of such glorious selflessness in 2006 when a friend—and not a particularly close one—gave me one of her kidneys. Perhaps altruism's most vibrant expression is found in good Samaritans such as Mark Thompson, the donor who was moved by a wife's poignant letter seeking a kidney for her sick husband. But our current altruism-only system has a dark side: It imposes coercion of its own by putting friends and family members in a bind. They might not want to donate, but they feel they must, lest their relative die or deteriorate on dialysis. This uncomfortable reality is masked when the option of compensation is foreclosed, but it is exposed when the opportunity to compensate organ donors exists.

Consider the examples of Hong Kong, Israel, and Iran. When "transplant tourism" from Hong Kong to mainland China became feasible, living donations dropped noticeably. According to the Israeli Ministry of Health, which covers the cost of transplants obtained abroad since 1998, there has been a reduction in living donations from relatives in Israel itself.[40] The same phenomenon transpired in Iran after 1989, when the country established a legal, regulated market in kidneys.[41] Many needy patients felt relieved, as did their families: A kidney that could be obtained from a stranger eased the burden on ambivalent would-be donors as well as on the patients themselves, especially older individuals, who were reluctant to ask their children to sacrifice an organ for their sake.

In the United States, all transplants are altruistic—at least in theory. In reality, sociologists have written, familial dynamics may involve guilt, overt pressure, or subtle threats aimed at would-be donors.[42] Motives abound. There is the "black-sheep donor," a wayward relative who shows up to offer an organ as an act of redemption, hoping to reposition himself or herself in the family's good graces.[43] Some prospective donors seek community praise.[44] For others, donation is a sullen fulfillment of familial duty, a way to avoid the shame and guilt of allowing a relative to suffer needlessly and perhaps even die.[45] Inevitably, the status of "donor," which by definition should include only those who act voluntarily, is a broad category under which are subsumed some reluctant, conflicted, or resentful individuals who give their organs, but not in the spirit of unconflicted generosity.

Complications of intimacy don't end there. The "tyranny of the gift" is an artful term coined by sociologists Renee Fox and Judith Swazey to capture the way in which immense gratitude at receiving a kidney can morph into a sense of constricting obligation. In their 1992 book, *Spare Parts: Organ Replacement in American Society*, the authors write, "The giver, the receiver, and their families, may find themselves locked in a creditor-debtor vise that binds them one to another in a mutually fettering way."[46] When bioethicist Cynthia Cohen claims that compensating donors "transform[s] what should be an act of altruism into a commercial transaction [that is] contrary to our basic social values," she appears not to recognize, as Fox and Swazey do, that less-than-altruistic sentiments, motivations, and actions can fall under the umbrella of social actions we call gift-giving.[47]

Nor, it would seem, has Cohen spoken with real-life surgeons. In his 1992 memoir, Thomas E. Starzl, the preeminent transplant surgeon, wrote, "I and others had seen . . . donation made as a reluctant sacrifice to someone for whom there was little or no affection. . . . If a prospective donor was deficient in some way, usually intellectually, the family power structure tended to focus on his or her presumed expendability."[48] This so troubled Starzl that he stopped performing live kidney transplants in 1972.

Organ donation reveals the many faces of altruism. Its happy public image as a warmly glowing act of selflessness is partially fiction, and the darker side makes one sympathize with Dr. Starzl's decision and long for the anonymity of a donor compensation regime as a benign way to ease the pressure on emotionally conflicted loved ones.

Does Donor Compensation "Vitiate the Gift"?

Opponents of compensation allege that it somehow cheapens or undermines the meaning of giving away organs for free. David and Sheila Rothman, historians at Columbia University, worry that market exchanges will weaken the human bonds that are otherwise fortified through altruism.[49] Nephrologists Gabriel Danovitch and Alan Leichtman express their great concern "that kidney selling would distort and undermine the altruism and common citizenship on which our whole organ donation system currently relies."[50] Sociologist Amitai Etzioni urges the postponement of paying for organs in favor of what he calls a "communitarian" approach "so that members of society will recognize that donating one's organs . . . is the moral (right) thing to do . . . it entails a moral dialogue, in which the public is engaged, leading to a change in what people expect from one another."[51]

Thus, in their view, the harm of reducing the intrinsic motivation of altruism outweighs the benefit derived from increasing the number of organs. The Rothmans find this problematic at the level of the family as well as at the level of the community (where deceased donations operate):

> Rather than donate and run the risks of surgery and future com-
> plications, family and friends might opt to purchase an organ;
> and if the market is as efficient as proponents claim, the pur-
> chased organ would be equally sound.[52]

As James Childress has put it, "Proponents of a system of organ donation often appear to suppose that pure altruism marks the donation of organs to the community for those in need and suspect that the presence of any other motives vitiates the gift."[53]

This position was shared by the late Charles Fruit, chairman of the National Kidney Foundation and the recipient of a kidney, who wrote in 2006, "Families decide to donate the organs of a loved one for altruistic reasons. Payment is an affront to those who have already donated."[54] His conviction has been echoed by Dorothy Hayes from Stamford, Connecticut, who says that, "as a kidney donor, I consider cash for organs an obscene proposal. . . . It was a gift to me to offer new life."[55] Similarly, Michael Bourne, a professor of English who gave a kidney to his uncle, has written that compensating donors would be "repugnant and wrong." As he put it,

> No one is more powerful than a man who is giving away some-
> thing of value and asking nothing in return. When that person
> is risking his life, this power is infinitely more valuable than
> mere cash.[56]

These are valid points—as far as they go. But they depend upon a fundamental conceit that is unjustified: Hayes and Bourne presume that other donors should derive the same meaning from the transplant experience as they did. There is no other legitimate way of looking at the issue. In other words, they would penalize innocent people languishing on dialysis and facing imminent death for lack of an organ because others are not as purely generous as they were. While such "altruism" is obviously a sufficient motive for some donors, it is equally obvious that it is not sufficient to motivate enough donors to meet the needs of the thousands of would-be recipients on the waiting list. Why should those people be left to die simply to preserve the sense of purity that other donors enjoy?

Virginia Postrel (the journalist who was my kidney donor) has taken Charles Fruit to task for his attitude. "The argument that paying organ donors is 'an affront' to unpaid donors is disgusting," she writes. "Are unpaid donors giving organs to save lives or just to make themselves feel morally superior? Even in the latter case, they shouldn't care if *other* people get paid."[57]

According to Dolph Chianchiano, senior vice president for health policy and research at the National Kidney Foundation, the NKF Family Donor Council (comprising families who have donated the organs of deceased loved ones) believes that compensating donors would "cheapen the gift"—that is, reduce the value of the organs they gave to the people who received them.[58] This is a dubious assertion—though it seems plausible that some might feel that way—but even if it were true, it would only be true for *those* families; the vast majority of recipients would still consider the organs precious beyond words. What's more, those families would still have a moral obligation to supply the (presumably) small group of patients who would accept only altruistically offered kidneys.

If a person declines to donate because the act now seems devalued in some way, then one has to question whether his intention to become a donor was really motivated by altruism in the first place; after all, truly selfless motivations would not be extinguished because others are enriched. What's more, under a regime that offered the option of compensation, donors like Bourne and Hayes would have bragging rights: *They* were the ones who acted out of generosity, not for material gain. This would enable them not only to retain but to amplify the "warm glow" that comes from performing acts of charity, and which some theorists consider a major motive for giving.[59] This distinction is obscured by our current system because it requires that all who give must do so without reward. Given the importance of "social signaling" through gift-giving—that is, of using a bequest to announce one's civic-mindedness or generosity—the opportunity to accentuate the distinction should be most welcome to individuals who seek to make such a social statement.[60]

Would Bourne and Hayes have retained their own kidneys if other people were simultaneously being compensated for theirs? They do not say, and it is implausible to think they would not have saved a loved one; but Fruit, in his leadership role in the National Kidney Foundation, apparently feared that if the families of potential deceased donors were "affronted" by the idea of compensation, they might refuse to donate. Polls, however, suggest otherwise: Most people are either attracted by the idea of incentives or unmoved one way or the other.[61] What's more, family members of deceased donors typically donate for an emotional purpose, such as extracting some sense and goodness from an otherwise incomprehensible sudden death, to guarantee a kind of immortality for their loved ones after death, or to enact a good deed.[62] It is illogical to suppose they would deny themselves these comforts because enrichment was available to others. Needless to say, would-be altruistic donors who are bothered by the idea of compensation could always refuse to accept the money, or could donate their payments to worthy charities, enlarging further upon their good deed.

Conclusion

"We can either preserve human dignity," warns the National Kidney Foundation, "or engage in a wholesale sellout to the laws of supply and demand."[63] If these are our only options for addressing the organ shortage, then the decision is easy: Maintain the status quo and reject campaigns for donor compensation. But this is a false choice.

The true dilemma is larger and more ethically complex. It is a tension between respect for the dignity of rewarded donors *and* the amelioration of patients' suffering. Many critics appear to ignore this tradeoff. They rarely speak of balancing the risks against the benefits. Indeed, one would hardly know that the urgent calls to make donor compensation legal have arisen for a powerful reason: to stanch the needless suffering and prevent the premature deaths brought about by the lack of organs.

This is because the critics have a far greater allegiance to abstract ideas about dignity and the visceral wisdom of queasiness than to actions that could avert needless misery. To be sure, virtually everyone involved in transplant practice and policy prefers that altruism be sufficient to inspire an adequate supply of organs.[64] But, sadly, as we have seen, it is not up to the task. Some altruistic donors choose to express their personal values by insisting that all would-be donors derive the same meaning from the act as they did— a perversion of the very spirit of altruism. Even the fulfillment of familial commitments can be contaminated by hidden agendas and resentments.

And as far as social solidarity is concerned, how can we possibly rely upon collectivism to solve the problem when so many people continue to suffer and die on dialysis?

Ironically, a system based on altruism-or-else fails to accommodate one of the most widely held values in the bioethics canon: autonomy. Individual freedom is enhanced when options are increased. This includes the freedom to refuse remuneration. Indeed, just as "dignity" is invoked as a reason to oppose donor compensation, it can be seen as a potent justification for supporting it, because compensation promotes vital features of human dignity as commonly understood: the advancement of freedom, the amelioration of suffering, and the preservation of human life.

As much as I decry their values and choices, the critics have a right to their moral commitments. Their views, however, must not be allowed to determine binding policy in a morally pluralistic society. A donor compensation system operating in parallel with our established mechanism of altruistic procurement is the only way to accommodate us all. Right now, the law forbids latitude. Tragically, there is no room for individuals who would welcome an opportunity to be rewarded for rescuing their fellow human beings; and for those who wait for organs in vain, the only dignity left is that with which they must face death.

6

Altruism and Valuable Consideration in Organ Transplantation

Richard A. Epstein

The present legal regime for organ transplantation in the United States was created by the National Organ Transplant Act (NOTA) of 1984, which includes an uncompromising prohibition of organ transplants performed for "valuable consideration."[1] With that prohibition, NOTA has enshrined altruism as the watchword of the transplantation establishment. Thus, the Transplantation Society proclaims, "Organs and tissues should be freely given without commercial consideration or financial profit."[2]

Unfortunately, the chief consequence of this policy choice is a persistent and growing shortage of transplantable organs. Even detractors of market transactions in organs grudgingly recognize that exhortation and other half-measures have not shortened the ever-longer queues for kidneys and other transplantable organs.[3] Not surprisingly, the growing kidney shortage has spurred demands for some liberalization of NOTA's prohibition by allowing, at the very least, a regulated market that provides some compensation for living transferors (who can no longer be called donors). According to Sheila and David Rothman, "The idea of establishing a market for organs, although certainly not new, is now attracting unprecedented support."[4]

Some proponents of compensation for organ transplants have urged that the government purchase organs at stipulated prices and then distribute them in accordance with standard United Network for Organ Sharing (UNOS) criteria.[5] Others, like myself, are willing to let prices vary freely in an open-market setting. Between these two positions are still other proposals that rely on tax or in-kind benefits (such as free health care to organ donors) to reduce or eliminate the current shortage.[6]

Nevertheless, defenders of the status quo raise a variety of ethical and practical objections to introducing any financial incentives. Their reform agenda stresses finding new incremental methods to increase the number of donated organs, whether through educational programs, the use of riskier (often infected) organs, or a redefinition of "death" (to include victims of fatal cardiac arrest as well as the brain dead) to expand the pool of organs for deceased-donor transplantation.[7] Opponents of incentive programs insist that their imperfections, evident in developing nations such as Pakistan and India, will be replicated in the United States.[8] They warn of the risk of transplanting diseased organs from paid donors who lie about their medical status to make the sale. And, finally, echoing the earlier work of Richard Titmuss on blood donations, they denounce paid transplants for impoverishing ignorant suppliers of organs and crowding out altruistic transactions.[9] It is possible even to point to cases of fraudulent refusals by transplant intermediaries to pay for harvested organs on the bald assertion that the organs were not of usable quality.[10] More philosophical critics fear that organ sales will lead to the commodification of the human body, a diminished respect for the voluntariness of consent, a compromise of individual autonomy, and a reduced level of emotional support within families.[11]

These objections are all overstated. None justifies NOTA's wholesale ban on organ transactions. Nor do they justify the large expenditures incurred in ineffective attempts to expand the organ supply within the NOTA framework.

This chapter explores the philosophical and economic weaknesses of the prevailing legal regime for organ transplantation. In it I examine the inconsistent attitudes toward altruism that characterize current legal policy, and consider the choice between regulated and unregulated markets, advancing reasons to prefer the latter. Next we give some estimate of the value of a serviceable kidney and the net social gains we can expect from allowing kidney exchanges. Finally, we examine and reject any claim that financial incentives are self-defeating because they will "crowd out" voluntary donations.

Our Uneasy Embrace of Altruism

No one can gainsay the nobility of altruism, whereby an individual displays an unselfish concern for the welfare of others. Indeed, there are doubtless many cases in which ordinary people have put the well-being of others ahead of their own. At the same time, the powerful forces of individual self-interest predict that, like other precious commodities, altruism will be in short supply in a wide variety of social contexts. Most organized markets choose some form of exchange, such as sale, barter, or hire, precisely to avoid excessive reliance on generous impulses in the organization of social life. Any moral preference for altruistic organ donation must still contend with Adam Smith's simple empirical estimation that altruism alone will not stimulate individuals to act for the benefit of others, except in family or intimate group settings. Here are Smith's familiar words from 1776:

> Man has almost constant occasion for the help of his brethren, and it is in vain for him to expect it from their benevolence only. . . . It is not from the benevolence of the butcher, the brewer, or the baker, that we expect our dinner, but from their regard to their own interest. We address ourselves, not to their humanity but their self-love, and never talk to them of our own necessities but of their advantages.[12]

Although we can quibble on details, Smith's basic message is sound, even prophetic: It is dangerous for a social system to rely on a laudable but unreliable set of motivations. Markets succeed because they rely on the prospect of private returns from voluntary transactions to sustain the operation of the overall system in the long run. Smith correctly spoke of butchers, brewers, and bakers. It would be wrong to extend his argument to husbands, wives, and parents, for altruism and sentiment play powerful roles in intimate settings. These observable patterns are just one vivid instance of the "kin altruism" that is a staple of modern evolutionary theory.

It is, therefore, not surprising that, with respect to a risky organ transplant such as that involving transplantation of a portion of the liver, typically the only persons willing to undertake the procedure are parents and other close relatives of the recipient.[13] Quite simply, as personal connections grow weaker, altruism inevitably declines. Of course, heroic acts of rescue and charitable assistance to the poor, bereft, and disabled remain.[14] But rescues typically take place in unstructured situations where the direct perception of peril prompts people to action, and charitable transactions involve only the gift of time or money. Kidney transplantation requires surgery. In 2006, Good Samaritan donors who offered kidneys to those next in the queue accounted for only 66, or 1.02 percent, of the 6,435 living donors.[15] As the events of the past forty years have shown, their numbers would not have been increased by any combination of private exhortation, social tribute, or moral praise.

There is, moreover, good reason to think that our internal biological instincts work against our willingness to donate organs, with or without compensation. Cutting open the body is an unnatural act to which all sentient creatures develop a strong natural aversion. Biological sentiments do not evolve nearly as rapidly as technology, which is why anesthesia must be administered to perform surgery on living organisms not biologically equipped to distinguish beneficial from harmful invasions. Alvin Roth has recently made the provocative argument that this "repugnance" often places real social restraints on voluntary transactions involving the body,[16] and it follows that any inbred repugnance to cutting open one person to help another should doom altruistic as well as paid transactions. There are scars in both cases.

Today's ban on organ sales, therefore, cannot reflect disgust with the surgical procedure, but rather repugnance at payment, which does not have any biological source at its roots. Indeed, as Roth recognizes, the common culprit is the fear of "coercion."[17] Yet with organ transplants this term is used in a near-Pickwickian manner that does not distinguish between the threat of a harm and the promise of a benefit. When, for instance, Gaston, Danovitch, Kahn, Matas, Schnitzler, and I advanced a modest proposal to allow a regulated market in organ transplantation,[18] Mark Fox responded that it was "coercive" to persons of limited means, and so reflected "the folly of the privileged, not the reality of the poor."[19] How the poor are hurt by an expanded set of options, Fox never explained. Clearly, we have learned to overcome our natural revulsion to surgery. It would help greatly if Roth and Fox criticized, rather than just recounted, broad definitions of coercion that condemn voluntary exchanges for mutual advantage as if there were a taking by A from B.

This drumbeat of coercion has also been directed at an organization called LifeSharers that seeks to expand organ supply.[20] Impatient with the current legislative logjam, its founder, David J. Undis, a retired insurance executive, has implemented a program of donations in which, by agreement, each program participant is given preference over nonparticipants in receiving a suitable cadaveric organ from another participant.[21] In effect, LifeSharers introduces a weak form of promissory barter among group members. Ironically, LifeSharers in reality only takes a leaf from the UNOS playbook, whose current protocol puts live organ donors at the head of the queue should they need organs (a preference that is conveniently not regarded as "valuable consideration"). Yet, once again, Fox and his coauthors condemn the "coercive nature" of LifeSharers' preferred-status mechanisms, insisting that they play on the fears of potential members that they might not get needed organs.[22] Expressing a similar hostility to other innovative strategies, Sheldon Zink and her colleagues condemn all programs that aim to expand the organ supply by financial means on the ground that they undermine the current UNOS structure, with its elaborate queuing procedures.[23]

Such shortsighted and misanthropic views emerge from a misunderstanding of how altruism works. At present, UNOS allows an individual to make a directed donation to any person he or she chooses, irrespective of position on the waiting list. But this policy does not satisfy many critics of UNOS, who think that a communitarian ethic should be followed by requiring every altruistic donor—living or deceased—to give his or her kidney to the first person on the list. I disagree. Not allowing donors to choose their donees goes against every principle of charitable giving. The best way to nourish altruism is to permit individuals to connect to whomever they choose. It hardly helps to condemn generous individuals for making gifts to the "wrong" people. What matters is the completed kidney transfer, not some refined discussion of whether a particular donor is selfish or generous. Without directed donations, many prospective donors will just keep their kidneys. Yet allowing a directed donation removes one person from the queue, thereby shortening it for everyone who remains. Directed donations let everyone gain and no one lose. They do not create some dubious loophole for UNOS to close.[24]

The establishment's hostility toward directed donations does not apply to transactions within families or between close friends. But it does brand altruism toward *specific* strangers as somehow unethical or unnatural or, worse, a cloak for some hidden—and illegal—benefit in cash or kind. Arthur Caplan, a University of Pennsylvania bioethicist, voices outright opposition to any gift between strangers: "It undercuts the ability of the system to get organs to those most in need and who have the best chance to survive. . . . It's not fair because it gives priority to people who can get attention."[25] The first point is misleading, because "in need" refers, perhaps, to those patients who are "most sick," but these are not the individuals who will gain the greatest number of years of high-quality life. All too often the actual recipients are the persons nearest to death. They are not, as Caplan suggests, the persons "with the best chance to survive." Nor does Caplan explain why getting attention is a bad idea, given that it can often serve as a rough proxy of one's determination to fight the disease, or of a family's willingness to help out in times of stress. Finally, public solicitations generate positive externalities: Greater media coverage can make more people aware of how donating organs saves lives, thereby increasing supply.

Such conscious efforts to *solicit* donations from comparative strangers by advertising on billboards, in newspapers, and on the Internet have, not surprisingly, emerged from the limited success of donations within families or between close friends. A website called MatchingDonors.com, established in 2004 to link prospective donors and recipients, has come under particular scrutiny out of fear that it can invite covert payment in violation of NOTA. Matchingdonors.com takes whatever steps it can to block any violation of the law. Even so, UNOS has criticized the website because it requires a fee for participation, which is said to "exploit vulnerable populations"[26]—yet another overbroad reliance on the language of coercion.

Why this criticism should be directed at Matchingdonors.com but not other fee-based services is difficult to fathom. Surely, it cannot be because of its listing fees, which are often waived for persons in need. UNOS also protests that the program favors those with the best "media skills," which both ignores the modest increase in supply generated by the advertisements on the website and again imbues the dysfunctional UNOS list with an undeserved normative superiority. Socially, it is desirable for Matchingdonors.com to redirect organs to persons who may have a longer life expectancy or greater productivity than those at the top of the UNOS list. An organizer of a similar web-based donor-matching program said of the program's success, "We're drawing a lot of people to donate who wouldn't otherwise. We're saving lives."[27] Rather than buck the trend, UNOS should join it by using its own databases to create a similar service.

Neither directed donations nor preferential rights, however, can do much to negate NOTA's prohibition against valuable consideration. In particular, egoistic forces will limit LifeSharers' benefits. LifeSharers has not brokered any transplantation, and for good reason: Persons with pure altruistic sentiments do not need to join LifeSharers. They can just give their organs away in life or at death. More importantly, the LifeSharers program is dominated by paired kidney swaps.[28] In the simplest swap, the healthy spouse in one couple, for example, is blood type A, and his or her mate who has kidney disease is blood type B. The situation is reversed in the second couple, where the healthy spouse is blood type B, and the sick spouse is blood type A. Neither spouse can help his or her mate directly by transplant, but allowing the transfers across couples is a form of barter that helps both. The two healthy transferors have, in effect, entered into two transactions: each healthy spouse makes a gift to his or her sick spouse, but at the same time each healthy spouse barters kidneys with the healthy spouse of the other couple. There is thus an exchange between couples and a gift within couples.

UNOS claims persuasively that these transactions do not involve valuable consideration—a fiction for which we should be grateful.[29] But we know that altruism is not the sole force driving them, because all four parties are put under anesthesia at the same time to be sure that none can renege. To be sure, the participants in paired kidney swaps are no less altruistic toward their spouses than those who are fortunate enough to make direct organ donations. Yet, however we characterize the arrangements across families, within families the immediate return dwarfs any remote benefit that LifeSharers could supply. Given ordinary self-interest, the urgent necessity to provide an organ right now to a loved one weighs more heavily than the prospect of getting an organ in the distant future from some amorphous pooling system.

Regulated and Unregulated Markets

Faced with the structural limitations under NOTA, it is no wonder that efforts to stimulate the supply of donor organs have not come close to what is needed to eliminate the current shortages. Even under the best circumstances, securing a steady supply is surely more difficult for organs than for the consumables of which Adam Smith spoke. There are lots of repeat players in standard markets, most of whom are reluctant to cheat on a single transaction if they might jeopardize a profitable long-term relationship. In the absence of permanent intermediaries, however, organ transplants are strictly one-off, high-stake deals. Once one kidney is gone, no sane person will sell off the second. The market has to be properly structured the first and, more critically, the only time around. The market for organ donation is thus elusive and decentralized, both for altruists and egoists. Over the long term, the legal system must motivate many individuals to donate, knowing that each can make, at most, a one-time contribution to any overall reduction in the organ shortage. It is not possible for a single rich donor to overcome the shortage by donation except, ironically, by altruistically providing funds to purchase organs from nonaltruistic persons.

The question is how best to fill the gap. The key choice is between a regulated market in which only the government can provide the organs at stipulated prices and an open market in which prices can vary with supply and demand. This choice divides critics of the current NOTA ban. Arthur Matas is perhaps the most articulate defender of the regulated market.[30] Politically, I support his proposal wholeheartedly, relative to the status quo under NOTA. Indeed, if government administrators set prices correctly, the scheme might eliminate shortages altogether.

Nonetheless, in principle, I believe this proposal comes off as second-best. Government monopolies have never worked as well as competitive industries because they cannot harness all the available information to set prices and quantity at the correct levels. State monopolies don't work for ordinary bread; why think they will work for kidneys, whose value is so much more difficult to assess, given that their costs and benefits are not, as critics of organ markets stress, easily monetizable?

Second, an organ transplant does not involve a simple sale that exchanges goods for money. Unfortunately, any transplant poses serious personal risks to the seller, so *both* parties must be assured that their participation will not lead to death, disease, or other incapacity—which is why third-party intermediaries, including brokers, may fill the role of the repeat players needed to stabilize this market. Nonetheless, Matas takes an uncompromising stance against their use:

Under the system advocated here, no other commercialization would be allowed. All legal allocation of organs and payment for organs would take place through the government or government-determined contractor. Currently existing prohibitions on private brokers and contact between the donor and recipient would remain in place.[32]

I believe this proposed prohibition is a mistake. In industry after industry, brokers more than pay for themselves, especially in complex transactions. Where limited capacity and undue influence are serious risks, the dominant legal rule allows a weaker side to back out of a transaction when it has not received independent representation.[33] Why fight the wisdom of the ages and force ordinary individuals—all first-time players who might be reluctant to enter the organ market without professional assistance—to fend for themselves in dealing with government monopolies? Paid brokers could expand the possible set of matches for potential buyers and sellers and provide standard-form terms on which to base these transactions. As repeat players with fiduciary duties, these middlemen could help protect the weak and the vulnerable. By advertising their services in legal markets, they would use their reputational capital to create an implicit bond against their own bad behavior and that of their clients. And, surely, we should let hospitals and transplant surgeons help with that task. A voluntary market would founder unless it could assure sellers (just as it must assure donors) that they are suitable kidney transferors.

Last, the unregulated market would be able to break free of the UNOS waiting list, which gives undue preference to persons for length of stay on the list. Most likely, the higher bidders would be the persons who stood to gain most from the use of organs. That result would hold even for persons of limited means, for they would be more able to attract assistance from generous third parties if they had better prospects for good health. Indeed, since it is easier to attract gifts of cash than organs, my prediction is that voluntary charities would enter this market to help individuals obtain organs even when they had limited financial means. The decentralized control of unregulated markets should outperform government monopolies, here as everywhere else.

Measuring the Benefit of a New Kidney

Given that financial incentives could lead to an enlarged pool of kidneys, how do we measure the potential benefit? A detailed discussion of financial accounting and the medical cost-effectiveness of transplantation as compared to dialysis under our current programs for end-stage renal disease is presented by Huang, Thakur, and Meltzer.[34] Here I consider, instead, the broad psychological and social benefits of receiving a kidney transplant.

Let us begin by looking at some of the essential elements of any global analysis. First, transplantation is cheaper than dialysis. Arthur Matas and Mark Schnitzler have estimated the net savings from kidney transplants at $94,000 for each successful graft, excluding the improvements in quality and duration of life for transplant recipients.[35] For this social calculation, the identity of the payer is irrelevant; it does not matter that the government pays for dialysis instead of the individual. But these monetizable costs only account for a small portion of the overall cost of kidney disease. The dreadful suffering of patients on dialysis is a social given.[36] Any estimate of the costs of living on dialysis rather than receiving a transplant starts with the shortened life expectancy of dialysis patients, which today averages around four or five years,[37] and must also take into account the impaired quality of the patient's life from this harsh and unrelenting procedure.

To be sure, some evidence in the happiness literature suggests that the mental well-being of persons on dialysis does not decline as much as healthy individuals would expect;[38] but there is a clear tension between the optimistic findings in that literature and the more somber state of affairs revealed by the actual behaviors of dialysis patients. Other studies report a far higher rate of depression and other psychological disorders. Self-reported kidney disease has also been associated with a threefold increased risk of attempted suicide in the National Comorbidity Survey.[39]

In addition, as many as 25 percent of the deaths of individuals on dialysis result from voluntary withdrawal from the program, usually among older patients with other complications.[40] The difficult task is to disentangle the relevant motivations. One possibility is that withdrawal is a form of suicide—a desperate act by a patient who can no longer tolerate the physical and emotional strain of dialysis. A second view is that it is a rational end-of-life decision made by composed individuals in consultation with their families. These patients are likely suffering from comorbid conditions, malnutrition, dementia, malignancy, pain, or physical immobility.[41] They might be ready to die. Data from the United States Renal Data Service suggest that about 1 percent of the five thousand to seven thousand voluntary withdrawals from dialysis in 2005 were suicides.[42] Kurella and others found that dialysis patients had an 84 percent higher rate of suicide than the general U.S. population, after accounting for differences in population distribution.[43] That result undermines earlier data in a 1971 study that found dialysis patients' suicide risk a hundred times that of the general population.[44] It also calls into question a landmark study of Scandinavian patients that found suicide rates among dialysis patients fifteen times those of the general Scandinavian population.[45]

Yet even these more recent studies do not resolve the question entirely because of the difficulty of classifying cases with multiple motives. The Kurella study reports all data in a strictly dichotomous fashion and does not seek to determine whether any of the cases that are tracked as withdrawal should be classified as joint causation cases, in which the question is how much being on dialysis increases the odds of withdrawal from treatment, relative to patients with roughly analogous conditions who are not on dialysis. That study, therefore, represents a lower boundary on the number of suicides attributable to dialysis; but given its methodology, it cannot capture all the cases.

The hard question is how much one should bulk up the number of suicides to take into account these partial cases. Here is one way to approach the problem. Kurella's data report that for all patients the number of suicides is 264, and the number of patients who withdraw from dialysis is 44,465. It is unlikely that many of the reported suicides were, in fact, simple withdrawals. People are reluctant to report deaths as suicides when they are not. But if we assume that 1 percent of the reported withdrawal deaths were attributed to suicide, the 264 becomes 509, so that the increment over the base rate is no longer 1.84 but 3.54. That number seems quite low. If one substitutes 5 percent, the new number becomes 2,487 (2223 + 264), or 17.33 times greater. And, ironically if one-third of the deaths are attributable to the dialysis, the level of increase is around 105 times. This last estimate seems high, to be sure, but the 5 percent incidence surely does not.

Even if the more optimistic happiness assessments are accurate, they necessarily omit the loss in individual productivity of the dialysis patient and the social stress that constant dialysis imposes on the patient's family and friends. Since no composite measure of the total psychosocial effects exists, let us assume for the sake of argument that the value of a year spent on dialysis generates, at most, one-half the satisfaction of a year of good health—a "back-of-the-envelope" estimation that is sufficient to allow us to conduct the following thought experiment.

Consider, first, the median value of $250,000 that Murphy and Topel place on a year of good health. The figure, which is derived from the amount of money a man in his mid-fifties would pay for reduced death rates from heart attacks and cancer, serves as a reasonable starting point for further calculations.[46]

The average patient starts dialysis at age sixty-two and survives for four to five years.[47] The Murphy and Topel figure translates into a psychosocial gain of $125,000 for each year spent on dialysis. From that figure, we must subtract the heavy costs of running a dialysis program. Huang and colleagues report that the total bill for dialysis in 2005 was $17 billion for about 314,000 dialysis patients, which works out to about $56,000 per patient per year.[48] To those costs must be added the other costs, both familial and social, incurred to care for these patients, including outlays by patients and families, which amount to about $4,000 per year. Together, these expenditures reduce the benefits of dialysis to $65,000 per patient per year. The present value of this income over the course of five years, discounted at the standard (inflation-free) rate of 2 percent is $306,375.

This is a substantial figure, but the net gains from dialysis are nonetheless dwarfed by those from receiving a serviceable kidney. A cadaveric kidney will remain functional for about eleven years; a kidney from a living donor will last about twenty.[49] Based on the average of these two figures, we can say that a kidney transplant provides about fifteen years of dialysis-free life to its recipient. We should not assume that living with a transplanted kidney returns the recipient to a perfect state of health, for complications may reduce the size of the potential gain. So a gain of $250,000 per year with a transplant sounds optimistic, but an 80 percent (or $200,000) estimate for restored health does not. To that figure should be added any extra earned income of the transplantee, as some studies have suggested that the employment rate of transplant recipients approaches twice that of demo-graphically matched dialysis patients.[50]

Offsetting the personal and financial gains from transplantation are its costs. These are far lower than those for dialysis. A plausible estimate places the cost for the first year of a living-donor transplant, including the one-time procurement process, transplantation, and postsurgical hospital-ization costs, at about $75,000.[51] The immunosuppressive drug regimen also imposes recurring, nonnegotiable expenses that average around $12,500 a year, reducing the annual gains of the transplant to $187,500.[52] The present value of this income over the course of fifteen years, dis-counted at a rate of 2 percent, is $2,334,237 after the one-time costs associ-ated with the procedure are taken into account. Subtracting the value of the five-year course of dialysis puts the present value of the net gains from the transplant at approximately $2,027,862. Divide that figure by two or four and the gains are still major. Whatever the difficulties in attaching dollar signs to psychosocial well-being, these numbers offer a tidy explanation of why so many people frantically search for kidneys for loved ones.[53] The gains are enormous.

The other side of the equation examines the cost to donors. Kidney transplants have become remarkably safe, with an anticipated mortality rate of about three persons in ten thousand.[54] The average organ transferor is around forty years old, with a life expectancy of about forty years.[55] Each donor death, therefore, results in the loss of about 2,080 weeks of life. Three such deaths equal about 6,240 weeks, which, spread over ten thousand per-sons, averages about four days of expected life per person—with obviously a very skewed distribution. Bicycle-riding and cosmetic surgery are riskier. Based on these calculations, the monetized value of the risk of the donor's death is around $5,000, to which must be added the costs of impaired func-tion, further health-care treatment, and any income loss from reduced employment prospects. Transferor complications are estimated at under 2 percent which, our Gaston group estimated, add costs of between $23,525 and $32,800 per transplant. This figure is probably low because it ignores personal anxiety, family tensions, and risk aversion from uncertainty. Let us put the total figure, then, at $50,000 or $100,000, which is large enough to make even dedicated altruists pause. And so the inability to find altruists who are prepared to sacrifice personal interests worth $50,000 or $100,000 makes it impossible to unlock $2.7 million of estimated potential gains. Perhaps these exact numbers are overstated. The relative magnitudes are not.

Crowding Out

There remains one last bastion of opposition to the use of financial incentives in kidney transplantation. Quite simply, the communitarian response is that such a program will prove self-defeating, since any increase in the number of paid donors will result in an equal or greater displacement of altruistic donations, as payment for organs "crowds them out." Sheila and David Rothman call such displacement one of the "hidden costs" of donor compensation. They suggest, as well, that it might "engender conditions inimical . . . to social cohesion."[56] Nephrologists Gabriel Danovitch and Alan Leichtman echo the latter sentiment in their article, "Kidney Vending: The 'Trojan Horse' of Organ Transplantation": "Our greatest concern is that kidney selling would distort and undermine the altruism and common citizenship on which our whole organ donation system currently relies."[57] It is important to examine the theoretical and empirical evidence that can be brought to bear on this question.[58]

Theoretical Concerns. The argument that compensation for organs will undermine altruism is a serious challenge to incentive programs, for if it is descriptively correct, then any such efforts will only intensify the already intolerable shortages. Fortunately, there is no reason to think that an organized market will have this effect in this context, any more than it has had in other contexts. The simple observation here is that one does not have to appeal to any considerations of social cohesion to explain the current shortages. Standard neoclassic economic theory predicts massive shortages when valuable commodities can only be sold for $0. The dollop of altruism shifts the supply upward, but it does nothing to undo the shortages. Why, then, reject the predictions of this simple model of how people would behave if financial incentives were allowed, when it already offers an accurate description of how they behave under the present NOTA ban?

To sharpen the theoretical argument, consider different variations on the basic crowding-out theme. One claim is that payments given to some will signal to others that they should refuse to participate in a system that refuses to honor their deepest preferences. But why? Charitable activities often take place side by side with paid ones. The true altruist should be more concerned with the condition of the potential recipient than with the financial motivations of other individuals who receive payment for their organs. With blood, for instance, the small sums paid might be construed as denigrating the gift, but the far higher prices in any anticipated kidney markets would dispel any such illusion, and they should help reinforce the undeniable fact that every kidney is precious.[59]

Even if we suppose that crowding out does persuade some altruists to leave the market, the next question is, how many will leave? We can be quite confident that close family members will not abandon a planned donation for a patient who cannot procure a kidney by purchase. If Jones receives $100,000 from Smith for an organ, Williams is not likely to let her spouse languish on dialysis. The only people who refuse to donate are the few who take genuine umbrage that others have accepted payment. But some of these potential altruists might remain in the market by taking cash themselves. And they are likely to be joined by a much larger number of healthy persons who enter the market for financial gain. Any transfer payment to lapsed altruists, moreover, does not count as a *social* cost, for the private loss to the payer is offset by an equal gain to the payee. What matters from the social perspective is the unambiguous increase in total supply.

Going further, let us suppose the supply response is so strong that individuals no longer give organs to family members, but choose to purchase them instead from third parties. Here altruism remains when the parent buys an organ for a child, just as it does when an organ is obtained today through paired donation. In addition, the ability to find a third-party organ supplier removes much of the unbearable social coercion that individuals can put on reluctant family members to become donors. Organ donation under the current rules is not nearly as romantic or selfless as the defenders of the current system believe.

There are other sources of gain as well. The person paid could be younger and healthier than the family member, or a better match with the organ recipient. If so, then the cash payment secures both a lower risk to the transferor and a greater benefit to the recipient, all at a modest transaction cost. The emergence of this market should, therefore, be welcomed as a general social improvement that leaves everyone better off and no one worse off. People who care more for the well-being of other individuals should laud, not condemn, these transactions. At the very least, they should welcome experiments to see whether the relaxation of the UNOS ban increases overall supply. If it does not, everyone will want to stop. If it does, then we should move to expand any program that enjoys some success.

Empirical Evidence. One cost of the NOTA ban is that it is impossible to gather direct empirical evidence as to how paid organ markets, regulated or unregulated, might work. Most of the evidence has to come from other sources. The one active market that supplies some information is the market in blood and plasma. The criticisms of that market made nearly forty years ago by Richard Titmuss in his seminal 1971 book, *The Gift Relationship: From Human Blood to Social Policy*, are said to offer compelling arguments against relaxing the NOTA ban. I believe that Titmuss misunderstood how markets operate and, in consequence, was far too pessimistic about paid transactions.

Without question, as Titmuss pointed out, a sale system may induce some desperate people to lie about drug abuse and prostitution in order to sell blood. But this risk presents a serious danger only when there is no independent way to screen blood for various conditions. Titmuss wrote a couple of years too early, for in 1973 sensitive tests emerged to detect hepatitis B, followed by tests for hepatitis C and HIV. Similar tests helped secure the blood supply from AIDS in the early 1980s.[60] In addition, Titmuss did not see the importance of payments to repeat suppliers of plasma, for which voluntary efforts at collection prove insufficient.[61] Only the extensive use of paid individuals makes it possible for the United States to maintain a thriving domestic and export business in blood plasma, almost all of which is obtained in exchange for payment. Since plasma collection is a much more time-consuming process than whole-blood donation, without remuneration there would not be enough providers.[62]

The overall moral is clear. Once the screening for contamination improves, safety risks can be handled directly. Once those safety issues are under control, cash payments can be used, if necessary, to increase supply, which varies from region to region, without creating an unwanted moral hazard. In any event, it is always possible to adopt a mixed strategy, in which certain people are forbidden to sell (or, for that matter, donate) blood, while others are allowed to either sell or donate, or do both, at their own choice. Reliable tests offer a far superior way to deal with health risks than an outright prohibition on blood or plasma sales.

Blood, moreover, is not readily comparable to kidneys. Under any legal regime, shortages of blood are far less likely than shortages of kidneys. The operational definition of an altruistic act is one in which an individual reveals unselfish motivation by taking an action that has a net cost to the actor in order to secure some gain to the recipient. But the level of altruism is sensitive not only to human motivations, but to the size of the expected sacrifice. Quite simply, pure altruism is less likely for kidneys than for blood, owing to the cost differential. The person who donates a pint of blood worth $100 is far less likely to donate a kidney with an implicit cost (as we calculated above) of between $50,000 and $100,000. Thus, the widespread, weak altruism of blood donations has not, and will not, be repeated for kidneys.

Conclusion

Clearly, the gains from trade are so great that the legalization of organ sales (or at least the use of valuable consideration in some form) should be allowed, subject to modest safeguards of the sort commonly used to prevent anyone from taking advantage of donors. The usual objections against financial incentives that prop up the NOTA ban are grossly inflated. The problems with foreign organ markets do not show the inherent weakness of such markets; they show only that no system of exchange can work without clearly defined property rights, strong contractual enforcement, and a range of intermediary parties who (as repeat players) can increase the confidence of potential transferors and recipients in the probity of the system. Altruism, however worthy, cannot trump self-interest as the dominant motivation in human affairs. Until we remember that simple lesson, we are doomed to suffer through the chronic shortages of organs that have developed in recent years. We must start down the road toward financial incentives, for otherwise the growth of the UNOS waiting list will continue unabated. Only liberalization of the organ market can prevent more needless deaths.

7

Crowding Out, Crowding In, and Financial Incentives for Organ Procurement

Benjamin E. Hippen and Sally Satel

Opposition to organ donor compensation based on fears of "crowding out" gathers empirical sustenance from an intriguing intersection of psychology and economics.[1] Drawing from an inference first offered by the late Richard M. Titmuss in his landmark 1971 study on blood procurement, *The Gift Relationship: From Human Blood to Social Policy*, motivation crowding theory challenges the premise that the supply of a good or service increases in response to an offer of monetary incentive.[2] Contemporary proponents of "crowding out" argue that, contrary to orthodox neoclassical economic theory, certain kinds of desired behaviors actually decrease in response to the offer of an incentive. Here we examine documented examples of crowding out to determine whether they support predictions that offering compensation to kidney donors would cause volunteer donation to decline so dramatically that the total number of available organs would fall below the precompensation baseline.

Blood Procurement: Richard Titmuss's Gift Relationship

Among the most influential contributions to the scholarship on the social milieu of blood procurement was the work of Richard M. Titmuss, a professor of social administration at the London School of Economics. Titmuss wrote widely about class inequality and was instrumental in shaping the British welfare state. In 1971 he published *The Gift Relationship*, which became a bestseller in the United States. The book ostensibly offers an empirical basis for the contemporary concern that offering incentives for transplantable organs might create the risk of crowding out altruistic donation. Reviewing the available data from surveys of blood procurement practices in the United States in the 1960–70s, where various forms of incentives (including monetary compensation) were offered to some blood donors, Titmuss concluded that less than 10 percent of all procured blood at that time was from truly voluntary donors—or, in Titmuss's taxonomy, "voluntary community donors" who expected no personal gain.[3] Contrasting this with blood procurement practices in the United Kingdom, where he found "99 percent" of donors to be of the voluntary community kind, Titmuss's work became the progenitor of the thesis that incentives serve to "crowd out" *authentic* altruistic donation.[4]

Titmuss's opposition to incentives was not predicated on the contention that they would actually reduce the total amount of blood available. The shortfall was concomitant with a rapid expansion in the availability and efficacy of multiple surgeries (cardiovascular and solid-organ transplant surgery) that drove the demand for blood and posed significant challenges to procurement organizations to keep up.[5] Titmuss did argue, however, that commercialization introduced inefficiencies into procurement practices, such as the hoarding of blood by individual hospitals, wastage of blood products, and geographic variation in a stable and available blood supply at any one time.[6]

Titmuss's conclusion that monetary and some nonmonetary incentives had a corrosive effect on altruistic donation inspired the U.S. Department of Health, Education, and Welfare to initiate a policy of promoting volunteerism in blood donation in the mid–1970s.[7] A closer examination of the methodological and moral assumptions at work in *The Gift Relationship*, however, raises serious questions about his thesis. As a number of economists have noted, Titmuss relied too heavily upon anecdote and incomplete data, rendering his portrayal of the U.S. system inaccurate in many respects.[8] By his own admission, Titmuss felt obliged to fill in a number of blanks: "There are so many inadequacies, gaps, and errors in the statistical data that at various points we have been forced to employ what one can only call 'informed guesswork,'" he wrote.[9] Part of this "guesswork" entailed making highly speculative numerical estimates of different sources of blood procured in the United States, in conjunction with further speculation regarding the motives of entire classes of blood donors.

An example of this methodological style was Titmuss's synthesis of the distinct categories of "responsibility fee donor" and "family credit donor." Responsibility fee donors were defined as people who received blood or blood products while hospitalized and were subsequently required by the hospital to "pay back" the blood, either by becoming donors themselves, finding others to donate in their stead, or paying the (high) cash value of the blood. Family credit donors each donated a unit of blood in exchange for insurance that would cover all their blood needs and those of their dependents for one year, an arrangement that could be renewed annually. Titmuss classified both "fee" and "credit" donors as nonaltruistic and reported that 52 percent of all blood procured in the United States from 1965 to 1967 came from individuals in one of these two categories.[10]

Titmuss permitted himself considerable latitude in assigning blood donors to these two categories. For example, he reported that 35 percent of the 6 million units of blood procured by the Red Cross in 1967 (which represented approximately half the blood collected that year) came from AFL-CIO factory workers through the union's community outreach program. Without further elaboration or obvious justification, he qualified this example of apparently altruistic behavior: "If the facts were known," he asserted, some significant fraction of this population would be responsibility fee donors or family credit donors, rather than the "voluntary community donors" he lauded elsewhere.[11] Thus, Titmuss's case that compensated blood procurement rampantly crowds out authentically altruistic blood donation rested on defining altruism as parsimoniously as possible, leaving the percentage of authentically altruistic blood donors meager, indeed. Despite stacking the deck in this fashion, Titmuss's own data undermined his thesis about the relationship between monetary incentives and procurement practices. Far from being the overwhelming source of blood procurement in the United States, purchased blood represented only 29 percent of blood procured, even during the heyday of compensating donors.[12] In contrast, since the United Kingdom had virtually no opportunities for blood procurement other than donation without strings attached, it is perhaps unsurprising that "greater than 99 percent"[13] of British blood donors qualified as authentically altruistic.

If Titmuss was stingy in classifying blood donors in the United States as authentically altruistic, he was considerably more generous in analyzing the conduct of his own countrymen. In an effort to provide a more objective assessment of the (rather tendentiously assigned) motives of American and British blood donors, Titmuss used a survey he borrowed from the American Red Cross to canvass the attitudes of the latter. His expressed hope was that data from this survey would be useful in comparing the (self-identified) motives of the two groups.[14] *The Gift Relationship* offered no comparison between the British blood donors he surveyed, however, and any comparable group of American blood donors. This omission is less surprising when one examines the two operative survey questions:

Q. 4: Please tick on the list below the *main* reason why you give blood?

(a) General desire to help people

(b) To repay in some way a transfusion given to someone I know

(c) In response to an appeal for blood

(d) Some of my friends/colleagues give blood and encouraged me to join them

(e) Another reason (please state)

Q. 5: Could you say why you *first* decided to become a blood donor?[15]

It turns out that, in his analysis of the British responses to the American Red Cross survey, Titmuss gathered answers (a) through (d) under the rubric of "voluntary community donors." The only way those surveyed could *fail* to be so categorized was to bypass the opportunity to choose from the offered menu of virtuous motives in favor of self-generating some less noble sentiment. Whether the answer to question 4 in some sense overdetermined the open-ended answer to question 5 was not considered, though the elicited answers to question 5 did uncover more nuance and complexity in respondents' behavior. Among the 26.4 percent of people whose open-ended answers were grouped under "altruism general and particular," the majority repeated or slightly rephrased choice (a) from question 4: "a general desire to help people." Titmuss tabulated other frequent answers under the categories of a "general appeal for donors" (18 percent) and "reciprocity" (9 percent), the second of which indicated a sense of obligation to repay blood given to the respondent or others; and more than 10 percent cited either reasons associated with the "war effort" or donation habits ingrained while in the armed services.[16]

Recognizing that this diversity of responses could not be gathered under a pristine definition of self-effacing altruism, Titmuss instead summed up the results as an extension of a communitarian concern among British donors:

> What was seen by these donors as a good for strangers in the here-and-now could be (they said or implied) a good for themselves—indeterminately one day. . . . In not asking for or expecting any payment of money these donors signified the belief in the willingness of other men to act altruistically in the future.[17]

One is left to ponder the irony: If Titmuss had been less obviously self-serving in his classification of American donors, and more self-effacing in his classification of British donors, his comparative analysis of the motives of donors in these two countries might have been considerably more subtle and interesting than it actually is.

As we have observed, British donors had no choice in how they gave blood, since the opportunity to engage in any kind of material exchange, available to some blood donors in the United States, was simply not an option. Under conditions of plenty, this arrangement was not generally problematic for the British. But under conditions of scarcity, the limits of altruism as an organizational principle of blood procurement became plain. When the need became acute for plasma products that were more difficult to procure, such as concentrated Factor VIII,[18] the flaws of the U.S. system of paid procurement seemed suddenly not so terrible, after all. As Douglas Starr relates, "Barely able to furnish enough whole blood, the [British] system proved incapable of marshalling an adequate plasma supply. . . . The nation's government-funded fractionation centers at Oxford and Elstree did not expand their capacities in time," with the consequence that the United Kingdom had to import more than half of its Factor VIII from the United States.[19]

Altruistic blood donation in the United Kingdom, then, was decidedly "crowded in," in the sense that any other means of procuring blood was illegal. But this system was only sustainable by aggressively, if quietly, patronizing the for-profit procurement system in the United States so as to remedy shortfalls in the supply of blood products such as concentrated Factor VIII. And, indeed, donor-only countries continue to be subsidized by the purchase of blood products from the United States—a $6.6 billion worldwide market in 2005.[20] Presumably, Titmuss would not have found it appealing to have to defend a system of altruism that was organizationally dependent on a thin veneer of hypocrisy.

From a psychological standpoint, Titmuss believed that the altruistic impulses of prospective donors were oppressed by the very existence of a commercial market. The simple knowledge that some might be paid, he speculated, suppressed the giving spirit in others by suggesting to them that they "need no longer experience a sense of duty, of obligation, of responsibility for strangers."[21] Famously, Titmuss framed his argument in the vernacular of "freedom," arguing that incentives for blood procurement infringed on the freedom to give blood to anonymous strangers. Donors, he argued, "should not be coerced or constrained by the market."[22] Prominent economists such as Kenneth Arrow have expressed bewilderment as to why Titmuss said "this willingness [to give] should be affected by the fact that other individuals receive money for these services."[23] Moreover, it is unclear how Titmuss could be so certain of a dynamic process at play—that is, the suppression of altruistic intent—when his observations were merely static comparisons of two systems. Titmuss lacked any meaningful comparison between conditions before and after commercialization to undergird his robust cause-and-effect claims regarding the introduction of incentives and subsequent altruistic behavior.[24]

At its best, Titmuss's empirical work reveals that the internal motives of British blood providers in the 1960s were nuanced and complex, even when the opportunity to give blood was crowded in by laws requiring donation alone. Had Titmuss been less hostile in characterizing the motives of U.S. blood donors, he might have more thoroughly developed a key insight of *The Gift Relationship*, a point elucidated more clearly by contemporary scholars: Even in a system where monetary incentives for blood procurement are prohibited, and donation is the only means available to provide and procure blood, donors have a plurality of motives, not all of which are coherently understood as "altruism." This is problematic for those who would claim Titmuss as a forefather in identifying the process of "crowding out." If multiple motives for donation are in play, then, first, there is no *necessary*, unwavering relationship between the organizational means of blood procurement and the specific motives for donation (that is, not all donors in a donor-only system are altruistic, and not all those taking incentives for blood are avaricious);[25] and, second, it is more difficult to make the case that *altruistic* motives are *uniquely* crowded out merely by the introduction of an opportunity to receive an incentive.

Finally, we should note that Titmuss also drew a connection between commercialization and the safety of purchased blood. In *The Gift Relationship*, he documented unacceptably high rates of post-transfusion hepatitis in the United States from contaminated blood. He inferred that paying for blood eroded a sense of community, and that a commercial system attracted blood providers who were less concerned about their fellow men and the quality of the blood they gave than they were about the payment they would receive.

It is true that many of the individuals who sought to be paid for their blood at the time of Titmuss's study were disproportionately impoverished, engaged in high-risk behaviors, and at high risk for being infected with hepatitis. But this turned out not to be a compelling reason to condemn a commercial procurement system, as scholars were able to show that poor-quality blood did not flow from the cash payment per se, but rather from the donor population to whom the payment was offered, in conjunction with inadequate screening techniques.[26] Some voluntary blood-collecting groups reported that their donors' rates of hepatitis B were as high as those of paying groups, while some blood collected by commercial groups proved to be as disease-free as the cleanest donations obtained by the voluntary groups. Socioeconomic characteristics of donors, such as income level and location of residence, were more strongly correlated with testing positive for hepatitis antigens than whether or not the donor was paid.[27] Other collectors found they could avoid tainted blood by setting up procurement sites in middle-class neighborhoods where most prospective donors were employed and owned their own homes.[28] Indeed, markers of social capital, such as higher educational level and being a stable, repeat donor, appeared to be the best predictors of uninfected blood.[29] One blood bank director was reported to have screened out undesirable donors by rejecting those who were unwilling or unable to give a home phone number.[30]

But the most important facet of the challenge presented by viral hepatitis infection in the blood supply was the lack of a reliable, reproducible test to demonstrate the presence of the virus in donated blood. Once such tests (for hepatitis and HIV) became widely available, the rates of transfusion-related disease transmission plummeted. Indeed, some hybrid donation-commercial blood banks actually reported discarding more infected blood products from their altruistic donor population than from people who had been paid for their blood.[31]

Furthermore, the emergence of HIV in the blood supply in the early 1980s made it painfully clear that altruistically donated blood was not guaranteed to be safer even if presumably high-risk groups were avoided. Indeed, most of the infected blood came from a most socially conscious group with a strong, reliable record of voluntary blood donation: sexually active gay men.[32] Another striking refutation of the assured safety of free blood was the scandal over France's HIV-contaminated blood supply in the early 1990s. Remarkably, French authorities *knew* the supply was tainted, yet allowed the blood to be used. It is perhaps an understatement to call this an affront to Titmuss's insistence that volunteer blood was safe blood.[33] Reliable, reproducible testing to identify and avoid transmissible disease proved to be far more important than identifying (correctly or not) the motives of the people who donated or sold their blood. As one commentator summarized the situation, "Safety is a matter of practice, not ideology."[34]

Today the quality of blood provided to medical centers is very high.[35] In 1973, sensitive tests for hepatitis B were introduced, and, subsequently, tests to detect hepatitis C and HIV became available. Furthermore, the United States maintains a thriving domestic and export business in blood plasma, almost all of which is obtained from paid individuals.[36] It is abundantly clear that the safety of blood used in the clinical setting is not determined by whether or not it is paid for. Nevertheless, the National Kidney Foundation still subscribes to Titmuss's findings. In testimony before a congressional subcommittee in 2003, the foundation warned, "Payments for organs could undermine the integrity of the organ donor pool as was the experience of paid blood donations."[37]

Other Examples of Crowding Out

Critics of a market in organs have cited other examples of crowding out to demonstrate how the introduction of a sanction (such as a fine) might paradoxically promote an undesirable behavior at the direct expense of a desired behavior, or how the introduction of a positive incentive to promote a desired behavior may seem to change its meaning or significance, rendering it less desirable than it was before the introduction of the incentive. We explore a few of these examples below.

Israeli Day Care Case. Historians Sheila and David Rothman amplified the concern that the introduction of incentives might result in fewer organs procured. Their arguments drew on a study of ten Israeli day care centers, undertaken in 2000 by Uri Gneezy and Aldo Rustichini, both pioneering scholars in the field of motivational crowding theory.[38] These private centers in Haifa operated on the understanding, not articulated in their tuition contracts, that parents were expected to pick up their children by a certain time, and that at least one teacher would have to stay late if they failed to do so. After a period of observation to establish control rates of late pickups, modest fines (U.S.$2.50 in 2000) for delays longer than ten minutes were introduced in six of the ten centers. Within a week, the number of late pickups in the fine group increased significantly compared to the controls. After the fines were rescinded, the rates of late pickups remained comparable to pre-fine levels. This finding led the authors to conclude that "a fine is a price"—in other words, a charge for exhibiting an undesirable behavior can be perceived as a payment for offered services rather than as a penalty for doing something wrong. In this instance, the fine was a *fixed* price, and one apparently well worth paying in the judgment of many tardy parents. The intriguing empirical point is that the introduction of a financial incentive in this instance (or, in the case of the day care centers, a financial *disincentive*) actually encouraged rather than dissuaded undesirable behavior.

From the results of this study, the Rothmans inferred that the "extrinsic motivations" of monetary gain from participating in a market in organs may "weaken moral obligations" and result in a "crowding out" of the intrinsic motivation of altruism, thus possibly reducing the number of organs:

> As Uri Gneezy, a professor of behavioral science at the University of Chicago School of Business, observes: "Extrinsic motivation might change the perception of the activity and destroy the intrinsic motivation to perform it when no apparent reward apart from the activity itself is expected." Although the case for the "hidden costs of rewards" is certainly not indisputable, it does suggest that a market in organs might reduce altruistic donation and overall supply.[39]

Note that Gneezy did not extrapolate from a scenario involving a penalty (the day care example) to conclusions regarding rewards; the Rothmans made that leap. Indeed, a closer examination of Gneezy's work undermines the Rothmans' conclusion. In the aptly titled, "Pay Enough or Don't Pay at All," Gneezy argued that *small* payments may result in poorer performance than no payment at all. His conclusion was that the relationship between the amount of payment and improvement in performance is not always linear, and that at low levels of payment, performance may be inferior. As applied to organ markets, this is not an argument against payment in general, but against payments too small to improve performance, as suggested by the title of his paper.[40] Elsewhere, Gneezy and colleagues expanded on the thesis: "Our results demonstrate that individuals contribute more when large repayments are feasible than when nearly no repayment is feasible."[41] Gneezy's data support an argument not against organ markets but against *price fixing*, whether the price is fixed at a small remuneration certain to fail as an incentive or at zero, which captures the current situation. If supply is reduced by a small, fixed reimbursement but increases in response to a larger reimbursement, Gneezy's data offer an answer comfortably within the lexicon of neoclassical economics: "Pay enough, or don't pay at all."[42]

Volunteer Work. Surveys and social psychology experiments have found that subjects are less willing to participate, or participate as strenuously, in a task they had already agreed to perform for free if it is accompanied by an offer of money.[43] In social science surveys, volunteers often express a sense that an otherwise acceptable or even admirable undertaking assumes a "taint" when a reward is offered, or that they feel bribed. One proposed explanation of this phenomenon is that payment deprives the actor of the chance to signal to others that he is a charitable or civic-minded person. Apparently, the greater the desire to be liked and well regarded by others, the less effective rewards will be.[44]

Kieran Healy has persuasively argued that the social expectations accompanying certain exchanges can shift when institutions and organizations work deliberately to shape the meaning of the exchange.[45] Perhaps an actor's need to behave altruistically can be fulfilled if the reward is specifically reserved for those most in need, for example.[46] Indeed, those put off by the fact that compensation is available to others would be wise to accept the reward themselves and donate it to a charity, thereby leveraging their altruistic impulses into helping even more people. As for the lost altruistic donors—those deterred entirely by the offer of the reward, and undeterred by the harm thereby visited on innocent third parties (that is, recipients)—there is some evidence that they can be replaced through recruitment of new donors who will accept compensation. This will only work, however, if, as we have discussed above, the original offer is made attractive enough to overcome any attrition from the altruist dissuaded by even the offer of an incentive.[47]

Relevance of Crowding-Out Examples to Compensation of Kidney Donors

Few real-world data exist to indicate whether the ability to purchase organs crowds out kidney donation from either living or deceased donors. The data from individual countries need to be interpreted and understood in the context of a multitude of cultural particulars, some of which may not be known. Kidney and liver procurement trends in Hong Kong, for example, clearly illustrate the difficulty of drawing general conclusions. One critic of compensation has attributed a decline in Hong Kong's rates of living kidney donation to the 1997 transfer of the former British territory's sovereignty to China, which made it easier to travel to the mainland to illicitly purchase organs from living vendors there.[48] Others have disputed this conjecture, citing the lack of change in the number of Hong Kong recipients who purchased kidneys elsewhere before and after 1997, the unchanged rates of organ procurement from the deceased, and an (unexplained) *increase* in the number of post-1997 Hong Kong living-liver donations, a procedure which is considerably more risky to donors than kidney donation.[49] In further support of the tenuous relationship between altruistic donation rates and the introduction of monetary incentives for organs, after the legalization of the sale of kidneys in Iran in 1988, the annual rate of (uncompensated) living donation remained stable at 11–13 percent.[50]

Presumably, the ability to obtain a kidney from a stranger eases the burden on ambivalent would-be family donors as well as on the patients themselves, especially older individuals who are reluctant to ask their children to sacrifice an organ for their sake. But if those organs are not immediately available, as would undoubtedly be the case in the early stages of a compensation system in this country, the sense of obligation to help loved ones would likely remain. Significantly, none of the psychological experiments by motivation-crowding theorists focus on an activity like organ donation, in which the beneficial effects are immediate and the stakes are life and death. What's more, these experiments focus on the question of whether people who are prepared to perform an act voluntarily will be less willing to do so if they receive payment. They do not address the question at hand: whether those willing to donate their own or their loved ones' organs would become less willing if *others* had the option of getting paid.[51]

As the researchers in this area stress, it is difficult to extrapolate from highly controlled psychological experiments to the messier business of real-world decision-making. The Israeli day care study and a hypothetical market in organs are obviously discrepant in that living kidney donation is a one-time event, whereas picking up one's children at school on time is a comparatively repetitive exercise with comparatively minor consequences (as can also be said of another instance explored here—giving blood). The behaviors in question in the day care study were embedded in larger social relationships straddling the line between business and education—features not present in the organ market.

In another study—this one involving labor markets—Gneezy and List highlighted observational differences between "hot" and "cold" decision-making, which distinguish immediate and considered reactions to a situation, as well as "adaptation" responses to changing situations.[52] Hot and cold decision-making may have implications for how organ donation and participation in an organ market are viewed more generally by potential participants, but here again there are presumably relevant differences between the psychological processes being studied by behavioral economists in the laboratory and those taking place in the real world. The methodological hazards of generalizing are only enhanced by an incomplete—even erroneous—understanding of the social and cultural assumptions at work, a point no less frequently overlooked in cross-cultural discussions of organ procurement as elsewhere.[53]

Impact on Procurement of Deceased-Donor Organs

Even if the total number of organs procured were to increase in response to compensation, would market exchanges result in fewer being procured from deceased donors?[54] The infrastructure required for deceased donation is considerably more complicated and more expensive than that for living donation. A successful system of organ procurement from deceased donors requires hospital resources in the form of large and well-staffed intensive care units,[55] readily available operating room space, medical personnel who are competent in identifying and medically managing potential donors, procurement personnel who are skilled in successfully soliciting grieving family members, and laboratory facilities capable of performing sophisticated serologic and immunologic testing in a rapid, efficient, accurate, and reproducible manner. Once the organs are procured, another system is required to identify appropriate candidates for them and ensure a fair, reproducible, and transparent process of allocation. Since the availability of deceased donors is unpredictable, this parallel system must also be manned and ready at all times. The costs of maintaining the infrastructure of a robust deceased-donor program are significantly greater than those of procuring organs from the living in a controlled fashion during daylight hours.

By comparison, a potentially plentiful source of organs from living vendors substantially reduces the need for the effort (and the expense) of making these resources available rapidly and continuously. Organ procurement from living donors can be done during the daylight hours with plenty of personnel around; donors can be screened and rescreened for transmissible diseases, which increases confidence in the safety of the donated organs; and the transplanted organs frequently function more quickly and with fewer postoperative complications than those from deceased donors.

These circumstances would seem to make a strong *prima facie* case for market organs crowding out deceased kidney donation, though this result would be tempered by a continuing need for organs not readily available— or available at all—from living donors, such as hearts, livers, and lungs. The concern over crowding out overlooks this difference between living and deceased organ procurement. When families decide to allow their loved ones' organs to be retrieved, they know that all viable organs will be taken, not just kidneys. There would be no logic in withholding the organs of the deceased simply because the supply of *kidneys* was enhanced through compensating living donors.

The Iranian experience supports this contention. Iran's donor compensation system, which was instituted in 1988 and is the only legal one in the world, is fraught with problems that prevent it from being a model we would want to emulate elsewhere.[56] These difficulties do not, however, bear upon the question of whether deceased and living donation can operate simultaneously;[57] and though some critics have alleged otherwise,[58] deceased organ donation has not been "crowded out" in the Iranian system by the existence of a ready supply of organs both donated and sold by the living. Prior to the year 2000, there was no legislative recognition of brain death in Iran. After brain death became legally recognized as such, rates of deceased donation in the country increased steadily, from 1.8 percent of all organs procured in 2000 to 15 percent in 2006.[59]

Furthermore, altruistic living organ donation in Iran has coexisted with the purchasing system since the inception of the program, representing 11–13 percent of all procured organs since 1988.[60] While it is plausible that rates of living related donation would have been higher and the path to deceased donation might have been achieved earlier in the absence of organ purchasing, the fact remains that altruistic behavior persists in the case of living related donation and flourishes in the case of deceased donation. Altruistic behavior turns out to be more resilient than its defenders suppose.

Conclusion

Motivation crowding theory offers an intriguing series of challenges to a proposal for a regulated market in organs from living donors. Unsurprisingly, different critics of organ markets have different behaviors or motives in mind when expressing the worry that a market "crowds out" altruistic donation. Some decry the loss of the "altruism" component while accepting the neoclassical assumption that demand will generate supply. Others argue that market incentives will so adversely affect the meaning of organ donation as to violate the neoclassical assumption. The evidence, as we've seen, is rather more textured and complicated than that, but it clearly does not support the assertions of critics such as Richard Titmuss or Sheila and David Rothman that the introduction of market exchanges simply reduces either a desired motive (altruism) or a desired behavior (donation/procurement). As Kieran Healy has observed, a crucial challenge for proponents of organ markets is to design a system that is sensitive to "the organizational effort and cultural work that go into making these exchanges socially acceptable."[61] A more robust elucidation of this challenge has been the purpose of this chapter.

8

Rethinking Federal Organ Transplantation Policy: Incentives Best Implemented by State Governments

Michele Goodwin

So what should we do, legislatively speaking, when altruism is simply not enough to satisfy the growing demand for organs in the United States? Organ policy has been largely unaltered over the past two decades, a period in which the population of people needing transplants has changed dramatically in size and nature. What might be done to bring federal law in line with current circumstances?

Over twenty years have passed since the enactment in 1984 of the National Organ Transplant Act (NOTA), which prohibited the use of any "valuable consideration"—payment in any form—as an inducement for organ donation. NOTA also designated the United Network for Organ Sharing (UNOS), a private organization, to be its contracting agency to oversee organ procurement and allocation in the United States. The NOTA prohibition on compensating donors has created profound problems, severely constraining the avenues by which desperate patients can pursue organs. Their only choices are to risk death waiting on a seemingly endless UNOS list, or gamble with the possibility of incarceration and fines by seeking transplant options outside of NOTA's narrow framework.[1]

The federal gridlock in organ procurement policy created by the prohibition on compensation is a matter of grave national concern, and a number of questions that have not been closely examined by policymakers demand thoughtful response. On other occasions, states have been highly effective laboratories for experimentation with innovative approaches to long-standing public policy problems. It is only natural to wonder at this juncture whether the federal government should allow the testing of novel state plans to procure more organs for transplantation. A simple amendment to section 301 of NOTA could permit applications for state-level waivers to the proscription on exchanging "valuable consideration" for organs. States granted such waivers would be free to develop pilot or demonstration organ procurement programs, which would provide invaluable information about the effectiveness of different approaches to this complex issue.

Origins of American Organ Transplantation Policy

Organ transplantation policy has not always been a matter of federal law; in fact, before NOTA, the federal government essentially left this issue to the states. The first policy effort to address organ scarcity in the United States was initiated at the state level with the enactment of the Uniform Anatomical Gift Act (UAGA) in 1968. The UAGA was a model law which, by the early 1970s, was adopted in nearly identical form by all fifty states and the District of Columbia. Its creation was spurred by the National Conference of Commissioners on Uniform State Laws (NCCUSL), which convened a group of highly esteemed individuals, recruited and appointed by various state governors, to draft an organ transplant policy. Chairing the commission was E. Blythe Stason, a professor of law and former dean and provost of the University of Michigan.[2]

Most transplant scholars and commentators suggest that the UAGA focused primarily on *who* possessed the authority to donate, and under what circumstances organ donation could be made. These observations are accurate but incomplete. To credit the UAGA and its drafters with only determining who could donate organs ignores the framers' intent. Led by Stason, the commissioners made strides toward considering incentives as a means of organ procurement by leaving the question open to individual state legislatures and, ultimately, the democratic process.

Although commentators differ on whether the omission from the UAGA of direct language on this point was intentional or an oversight, there are indications that leaving the question of incentives for states to decide was reasoned and deliberate. As a dean, provost, and commissioner, Stason was known for being meticulous, methodical, and purposeful in the examination of ideas and the implementation of policies.[3] If the framers intended to ban the sale of organs, with Stason at the helm of the commission, they would have done so. But, Stason observed at the time, the commissioners felt that "the matter [of payments] should be left to the decency of intelligent human beings."[4]

After presenting the model law to their home states for ratification and enactment, legislators sought to work within the spirit of the original draft. Thus, in a radical shift, states that had previously enacted laws to ban payments for organs and body parts—among them Massachusetts, Delaware, Hawaii, Maryland, and New York—*repealed* those regulations.[5] In so doing, they, too, were expressly leaving open the question of incentives, payments, and other forms of valuable consideration, at least for the posthumous disposition of organs and human tissues.

Stason himself said that the UAGA drafters contemplated incentives and supported allowing states the flexibility to decide those matters. In interviews and writings after the enactment of the UAGA, the commission chair remarked that the question of payments was intentionally left open for states to decide.[6] Demonstrating a nuanced view of what organ transplantation in the United States would become, Stason acknowledged that the possibility of donors demanding payments might arise, but he did not hold that all payments would be unethical, immoral, or illegal.[7]

Federalism and Organ Transplantation

For the next sixteen years, the 1968 UAGA as adopted by the states was the only law governing organ transplantation in America. In devising a national policy on organ transplants in the 1980s, the federal government did not initially set out to change the UAGA's tacitly open position on incentives. In fact, early drafts of NOTA were silent on payment for organs; they focused, rather, on the creation of a nationwide procurement and distribution system. The restriction on payment or in-kind exchange for an organ was prompted as an afterthought and due, almost entirely, to the activities of one man: a physician named H. Barry Jacobs, of Reston, Virginia.

In the fall of 1983, Jacobs, whose medical license had been revoked five years earlier on a conviction for Medicare fraud, was making plans to establish an organ brokerage called the International Kidney Exchange. According to a 1985 account in the *Virginia Law Review*, "Jacobs intended to solicit healthy individuals to sell one of their kidneys at their chosen price. A person needing a transplant would pay for the cost of the kidney plus $2000 to $5000 for Jacobs' service" to, as the *New York Times* put it, "escape the tyranny of dialysis."[8] Prior to his emergence on the scene, there had been no evidence of commerce in transplantable organs in the United States.[9]

In November 1983, Jacobs presented his plan to a House of Representatives subcommittee chaired by Representative Al Gore Jr., at a hearing entitled *Procurement and Allocation of Human Organs for Transplantation.* His testimony was not well received—Jacobs's pugnacious manner could not have helped his cause—and he became the lightning rod for a general outcry against the idea of paying for organs.[10] Section 301, a provision prohibiting payment, was soon inserted into the draft bill.[11] It stated, "It shall be unlawful for any person to knowingly acquire, receive, or otherwise transfer any human organ for valuable consideration for use in human transplantation if the transfer affects interstate commerce." Violators could be fined up to $50,000, imprisoned for as long as five years, or both.[12]

NOTA proponents may have believed that the law left open many possibilities for states. But such an assessment would have been misleading. To the essential question—what powers do local governments retain to craft organ transplantation policies that respond to local dynamics and needs?— NOTA did not provide an answer, except in the negative. It made clear that certain authority was removed from states and citizens, prohibiting the legal implementation of any incentives or "valuable consideration" (an ambiguous term, which broadly included anything thought to generate financial and even *emotional* value) in local organ transplant policies. After 1984, state programs to offer individuals any sort of incentive for donating their organs risked running afoul of federal law.[13]

The federal move to ban all forms of "consideration" was a radical step, not in what it specifically entailed—banning payments—as individual states could have enacted such measures (as Virginia had[14]); but because it significantly removed autonomy at the state level by extensively encroaching upon state authority. In fact, states had collectively addressed organ transplantation before the federal government's involvement by ratifying the UAGA. Shortly after NOTA, the UAGA was redrafted to comply with the new federal law. By that time, however, Stason had died. The vision of the 1968 UAGA was gone,[15] and states no longer had the opportunity to consider incentives.

Transplantation after NOTA

Federal intervention in organ transplantation through NOTA has had several consequences. As the critical shortage of organs in the United States has worsened, attempts to enact responsive legislation to address the need for them have largely failed or been indefinitely stalled. UNOS now holds a monopoly on legitimate organ procurement, controlling not only how organs come into the transplant system, but also the criteria for who receives them. While the benefits of UNOS, such as its capacity to collect data, are clear, its drawbacks include a lack of efficiency and effectiveness in meeting procurement goals and a pernicious national system of organ rationing.

Perhaps the most problematic result of NOTA, however, has been the disturbance of a fine balance between Congress and the states in developing transplant policy to respond to circumstances that inevitably are experienced more intensely at the local level. Local governments and patients are bound to an antiquated and chaotic organ procurement system and left with very few options for experimentation with different approaches to solving this problem.

Pennsylvania is the only state that has challenged NOTA's ban on valuable consideration in any way. In 1994, the Pennsylvania legislature passed the Burial Benefit Act, which provided modest reimbursement of hospital or burial expenses of deceased donors—expenses that would have been incurred whether or not the organs of the deceased were retrieved. The burial act was intended as a "thank you" to the families of deceased donors, state authorities said, but, clearly, it could also have served as an incentive for family members to give permission for retrieval of a loved one's organs because the benefit here inured to them.[17]

The act also established the Organ Donation Awareness Trust Fund, all contributions to which are voluntary.[18] It authorized use of 10 percent of that fund to defray medical or funeral expenses of the deceased, with an upper limit of $3,000 for any one family, although at the time of creation the fund was only large enough to offer $300 to each family of four hundred anticipated donors.[19] From 1994 to 1999, the Pennsylvania legislature invested significant financial and community resources in studying whether this new law would conflict with federal law.[20]

The plan stalled, however, in the final stage—all that it lacked was a signature from the state secretary of health—over concern that the funeral benefit was a violation of NOTA's prohibition on "valuable consideration" for organs.[21] A state representative sought clarification from the U.S. Department of Health and Human Services (HHS) in December 2000 regarding whether reimbursement of donor funeral expenses violated federal law, but was told that HHS could not provide a determination and he should consult the Department of Justice for a definitive interpretation of Section 301, a criminal statute.[22] There is no evidence that this was pursued. In the end, Pennsylvania state legal department decided not to test the limits of NOTA by offering incentives for deceased donation and instead directed the funds intended for incentives away from funeral expenses for the deceased and toward reimbursement for food, travel, lodging, and lost wages incurred by living donors—costs already authorized under NOTA.[23]

A Pragmatic Return to the States

The federal government already has considerable experience with waiver programs. Indeed, some of most generously funded federal programs incorporate state waiver provisions, including the No Child Left Behind Act and the Social Security Act.[24] In the latter case, section 1115 grants authority to the secretary of the U.S. Department of Health and Human Services to waive specific requirements, allowing greater flexibil-ity for states to meet the needs of recipients in the Aid to Families with Dependent Children (AFDC) program and to balance those needs with state interests. The waivers also enable states to implement pilot programs and experiment with existing projects that promote the purposes of the AFDC program.

During the peak years of welfare reform, between 1993 and 1996, the HHS approved welfare waivers in forty-three states. According to the department, the projects resulting from the waivers ranged from "modest demonstration projects, limited to a few counties," to others that promoted "dramatic statewide changes in the AFDC program."[25] These waivers constituted the first wave of welfare reform in the United States, as "many of the concepts included in state waiver requests were later incorporated into the Personal Responsibility and Work Opportunity Reconciliation Act (PRWORA) of 1996."[26]

Wisconsin was a trailblazer in the use of waivers for welfare reform. Between 1987 and 1997, then governor Tommy Thompson cut the welfare caseload by 60 percent, far exceeding the effects of the robust economy and low unemployment that marked the decade.[27] Other states were inspired by Wisconsin's success and used waivers to transform their welfare rolls.

Beyond providing freedom from federal strictures, waivers also generate policy knowledge, as different states approach reform with different strategies. In June 2006, for example, HHS granted waivers to five states to tailor their child welfare programs.[28] One, Michigan, is concentrating on greater investments in early intervention services. The waiver to Virginia allows federal foster care funds to pay monthly subsidies to families who assume legal guardianship of children, removing them from state custody.[29] Iowa is creating a managed-care demonstration project that focuses on providing services and support to special-needs youths between the ages of eleven and sixteen so they can stay in their own homes.[30]

In the case of welfare, states were granted waivers to experiment with reform because the problems with the federal welfare laws were widely recognized, and the states were demanding the freedom to act. The question is whether any such demand exists today for state experimentation with organ policy. If states were granted waivers from NOTA, would they use them? It is hard to say, but there is at least some evidence of interest.

In Wisconsin in 2003, for example, state representative Steve Wieckert, with the support of the transplant community, introduced a bill allowing donors to claim a $10,000 state tax deduction to cover lost wages and expenses for travel, lodging, and medical care incurred by organ donors.[31] The result was the first tax incentive law for organ donation in the country.[32] The proposal of similar laws by two dozen states in the less than five years since then, with more than a dozen adopting them, suggests that the desire to experiment is widespread.[33]

Model Waiver Language for NOTA

Because the federal government has limited how states might sensibly meet organ demand at the local level, the best—and seemingly only—way, as long as NOTA is in effect, would be to allow them to waive out of the act by way of demonstration projects. Much can be gained by the use of waivers, nationally as well as at the state level, by decreasing the national waiting lists for organs and reducing federal costs. The goal would be to move patients from very costly subsidized dialysis treatments to organ transplants, which not only would save millions of dollars each year but would also promote better health outcomes for sick patients.

If the federal government wanted to empower states to experiment with different approaches to solving the organ crisis, how could it be done? Granting them waivers from the National Organ Transplant Act would be surprisingly simple. Section 301 of NOTA could be amended with language enabling them, as follows:

(a) *In order to receive federal approval for waivers of the provisions of the National Organ Transplant Act, states must demonstrate a negative impact of the current legislation. A negative impact can be demonstrated by chronic organ shortages in the state, extended waiting-list times, disparate impacts on selected categories of persons, such as the elderly or children, or other conditions that limit the states' ability to meet the needs of potential organ recipients.*

(b) *Waivers can be implemented for three-year periods and are renewable based on need and subject to approval by the secretary of health and human services. At the termination of the waiver provision, states are required to submit a detailed report outlining the successes of and obstacles to their programs. States must also provide a financial analysis to help assess which programs more effectively met the needs of citizens and reduced the costs associated with transplantation.*

(c) *States will be responsible for collecting, aggregating, and analyzing organ transplant data for waiver projects. Data collection should be based on models currently in use by UNOS, which specify donors by categories of living and deceased, but it should also be expanded to include specific classes of donors that result from pilot projects, including paired donors, directed donors, reimbursed donors, and others.*

(d) *States are not required to participate in waiver programs. Those that choose to participate in pilot projects shall be required to submit waiver applications to the secretary of health and human services. To receive approval for waivers, states must be willing to conduct rigorous evaluations of the impact of their demonstration programs. States may, for example, be required to assign patients on the waiting list randomly to control groups or experimental groups that are subject to the waiver. Equally, states may be required to track donors among the different donation categories.*

(e) *States may be required to track and compare success rates among different categories of donors and recipients. Success is defined as receiving an organ transplant. States may postpone until the waiver expires implementation of future federal organ procurement legislation to the extent that such rules are inconsistent with ongoing waiver provisions and protocols. States may choose to maintain or extend waivers to continue monitoring or evaluating their programs without a showing of further negative impact. States may apply for waivers and later choose not to implement the waiver programs without penalty.*

(f) States are required to show that waivers are cost-neutral, but only over the life of the waiver, rather than each year. "Cost-neutral" shall be interpreted to mean that costs do not exceed state and federal contributions prior to the waiver implementation. Waivers may be reapproved for three-year increments over the life of the waiver program. Termination of the program shall be subject to congressional determination. Waivers are subject to the approval of the secretary of health and human services.

Four principles would guide experimental programs made possible by the model waiver: saving lives; promoting better information collection and sharing; enhancing organ donation efficiency by providing as many options as possible to link patients with healthy organs; and improving cost-benefit ratios. The model encourages the development of strategies to reduce overall state and federal expenditures in the renal failure area by moving sick patients from dialysis to transplant, thereby enhancing survival rates while bringing down overall costs and maximizing the effectiveness of fund allocation. The language provides flexibility to states in the creation of programs while promoting consistency in data collection by basing it on models currently in use by UNOS.

The model waiver also attempts to address the very concerns that led to the enactment of NOTA—namely, that rogue opportunists might attempt to exploit the poor, circumvent legislative protocols, and otherwise undermine the dignity and legitimacy of the transplant system. States that wish to participate in the waiver program must demonstrate a negative impact of the current federal legislation. Although the threshold for doing so is high, most, if not all, states already meet the standard with chronic organ shortages, extended waiting-list times, or disparate impacts on selected categories of groups, any one of which conditions would sufficiently demonstrate that the intended goals of NOTA are not being reached. The model waiver promotes accountability as well, with its three-year implementation periods, renewable only based on indicated need and application to the secretary of health and human services. Requirements to supply data evaluating the success of the program and a financial analysis at the time of expiration hold a state further accountable.

The language of the model waiver could be applied to any of a variety of state organ procurement programs. While programs need not be incentive- or market-based, waivers are intended to free states to follow those objectives if they so choose. Pennsylvania's Burial Benefit Act, for instance, would have fit the waiver model. Interested states would probably elect to implement their waivers on a pilot basis, with funds for a compensation program coming from state revenues or supportive private sources, such as charities or foundations. Federal contributions might be feasible as well. Specifically, savings to Medicare from patients exiting dialysis could be passed on to the states through an arrangement called gain-sharing, in which hospitals and physicians can receive a portion of the savings they generate for Medicare through creative deployment of federally funded health-care resources.[34]

Such pilot programs would also generate information about donor compensation that the current national organ procurement system completely lacks. Those who suggest that incentives will never reduce waiting lists, or that they will exploit the poor, or that they will cause "crowding out"—meaning altruistic organ donation will go down if alternative models are introduced[35]—cannot prove their claims because they lack evidence. Equally, economists who have long suggested that introducing incentives into transplant regimes will likely save lives and dramatically reduce waiting lists have little evidence to support their contentions. The model waiver attempts to remedy this deficiency by promoting—indeed, mandating—data collection, which is crucial to the overall health of any procurement system.

Finally, the model waiver responds to the demands and concerns that emerge from the geography, demography, and values of each state. Conceivably, the trigger for organ-sharing lies outside of markets but is not quite met through traditional modes of altruism. Perhaps religion matters in these discussions, or values such as trust and confidence in the local procurement network. The best and only way to find out is to allow states to become laboratories of democracy for organ transplantation. Granting waivers to federal law that allow states to experiment is the best possible example of collaborative federalism.

Conclusion

Sally Satel

Let us return to *The Big Donor Show*, which aired on Dutch television in June 2007 and was described in the introduction to this book. Three days after watching what turned out to be a hoax—in the end there was no terminally ill young woman planning to bequeath a kidney to one of three desperate patients—over fifty thousand people downloaded an organ donor registration form from the Internet.[1]

This was surely a welcome development; yet, as the Dutch themselves recognized, more was needed. Several weeks after *The Big Donor Show*, the Dutch health minister solicited guidance from a national advisory body, the Center for Ethics and Health, on the ethical permissibility of incentives to donate organs.[2] In November 2007, the center's report, *Financial Incentives for Organ Donation: An Investigation of the Ethical Issues*, was released. Its authors concluded that "offering rewards for organ donation can be morally justified," and they proposed lifelong payment of health insurance premiums as motivation for prospective donors.[3] The director of the Dutch Transplant Foundation, Bernadette Haase, was intrigued by the recommendation. "If it is properly run and well organized, it could be a solution," Haase said.[4] In late 2008, the Dutch health minister directed health insurers to reduce annual fees by 10 percent for registered organ donors.[5]

Other countries have been exploring initiatives, as well. In Saudi Arabia, for example, the cabinet passed a law to compensate unrelated living donors with lifelong medical care.[6] The Indian government announced plans in early 2008 to amend its organ transplant law to offer benefits to the families of deceased donors, including health and life insurance.[7] The Ministry of

Health of Singapore expressed openness in the summer of 2008 to the idea of compensation: "By forcing ourselves to think about unconventional approaches, we may be able to find an acceptable way to allow a meaningful compensation for some living-unrelated kidney donors, without breaching ethical principles and hurting the sensitivities of others."[8]

As of this writing, Iran remains the only country with a legal system of donor compensation that offers a model with real benefits to the recipient but also significant flaws. It remains to be seen whether the Dutch minister will follow the recommendations he solicited, whether the Saudi law will be enacted, whether India will follow through on its announcement, or whether the "sympathetic approach" of Singapore's Ministry of Health will translate into a legal market. One thing is certain: Wherever we find openness to reform and actual attempts to innovate, we find thinkers and leaders who are able to envision a promising middle ground between the status quo—a procurement system based on the idealism of selfless altruism side by side with the dark, corrupt netherworld of organ trafficking.[9]

This book has illuminated that middle ground. It has shown how an ethically sound, medically safe, and economically rational program of donor compensation could be constructed to increase the supply of kidneys. It has done so by posing serious analytic challenges to, if not outright refutation of, the three key objections to donor compensation.

In answer to the objection that donor compensation is inherently wrong, the authors have shown, to the contrary, that appeals to human dignity form a more potent justification for promoting material incentives to donation than they do for rejecting it. If sincere qualms persist, we hope the book will help our critics tolerate their reservations and cease their campaign to block trials from even taking place. Enlarging the policy arena will allow donors of all different minds to discharge their moral commitments.

In answer to the objection that organ compensation, while not fundamentally unethical, cannot be implemented without exploiting the vulnerable, we have shown just the opposite: how a careful, donor-centered system can be devised, and how it need not be a "zero-sum game in which any advantage to one participant necessarily leads to disadvantage," as one vocal detractor has insisted.[10] At the same time, we have exposed the false choice put forth by critics, such as the physician who asks, "What sort of organ transplant program do we want—one that pressures the financially vulnerable with cash incentives, or one that encourages the show of kindness through a loving, voluntary gift of organ donation?"[11] A better question is this: "What sort of organ transplant program do we want—one that remains unresponsive to a growing public health disaster, or one that pursues ethically responsible ways to save lives and suppress the international organ trade?" The answer is that we must want a system that responds wisely to the disaster.

In answer to the objection that fewer people will donate freely if compensation is made available to donors, leading to an overall reduction in kidneys for transplantation, we have shown the serious weakness in the evidence that is purported to support this prediction. Meanwhile, virtually every known rule of social psychology and economic behavior contradicts it.

This book has accomplished its major goals of presenting the rationale for reform and presenting a blueprint for policy change. Meanwhile, it has deflated critics' alarmist predictions, illuminated their faulty reasoning, and revealed their intransigent refusal to join with reformers and help forge solutions that would address their most pressing concerns.

The Politics of Transplant Policy Reform

In these final pages, I will describe the political considerations that surround efforts to revise transplant policy.

What Should Congress Do? As Michele Goodwin has highlighted in her chapter, the states can serve as fertile laboratories for reform. A state-based model of reform is probably superior to a single policy emanating from the federal government. The latter is too risky. If a universal policy were not executed thoughtfully and failed as a result, this could be held up by critics as "proof" that no program of compensated donation could work. Multiple concurrent experiments across the country afford the greatest promise for flexibility and success. The waiver model proposed by Goodwin would enable states to experiment with incentives, yet not violate the prohibition against "valuable consideration" in the National Organ Transplant Act. It is a sound idea, yet it leaves a problematic law intact.

Perhaps an even more efficient and basic move by Congress would be to amend NOTA and change the very definition of the term "valuable consideration." As currently written in law, the term excludes "reasonable expenses" incurred by the living donor, such as travel costs and lost wages. An amendment should extend exclusion from the definition to any material benefits provided by federal, state, or local government to an organ donor. Such a revision would create no imposition or burden. It would simply open the door to states to experiment. Presumably, states such as Wisconsin and Pennsylvania, which have track records of creativity in this arena, would take the lead.

Implementation. Under this proposed revision of NOTA, a state could offer an incentive to an individual to donate a kidney to another resident of the state. In a streamlined system, prospective donors could make contact with a designated transplant center in the state, which would be the entry point for applying to be a compensated donor. A template for intake, follow-up medical care, insurance, and long-term monitoring could be based on the one suggested by David Cronin and Julio Elías. If the donor met all eligibility requirements, including the provision of informed consent, the center would find the best-matched transplant candidate within the state using the UNOS computerized system (UNet).[12]

The compensated donor would be offered the alternative of participating in a donor chain, in which the donor's kidney would go to a patient who had a willing but incompatible donor. That willing but incompatible donor could then give his kidney to someone compatible with him; and that recipient's donor could offer his organ to someone else; and so on and on, thus gaining the most possible benefit from the effort of each donor in the chain. Within big states such as California, New York, or Texas, the database of transplant candidates probably contains hundreds of such incompatible donors.

States might decide to offer a tax credit, state university tuition voucher, retirement contribution, health insurance, or other inducement. In an effort to expand the pool of cadaver organs, they might decide to reward the estates of the deceased or offer a generous funeral benefit to their loved ones. Some states might choose to pursue incentives for deceased donation only, viewing this as an intermediary step leading to the compensation of living donors. (They would save themselves any debate over exploiting the poor, but would almost surely procure fewer organs than states that rewarded living donors.)

The value of incentives for living donors would probably range between $25,000 and $40,000; less for the deceased. Funding to underwrite incentives could come from gain-sharing with Medicare, as described by Goodwin. Under such an arrangement, hospitals and physicians could receive a portion of any savings they generated for Medicare—in this instance, the savings that came from patients' leaving the dialysis rolls. If the patient were supported by Medicaid—a federal entitlement program administered by each state but funded jointly by the federal and state governments—then the saving to the state would be direct: It would no longer pay its share of dialysis costs. Incentives could also be underwritten by charities, foundations, or insurance companies.

Within such a framework, altruistic donation would continue in parallel with a system that offered compensation. Any medical center or physician that objected to the practice of compensating donors could simply opt out of performing transplants with organs relinquished by compensated donors. Recipients on the list would be free to turn down a paid-for organ and wait for one given altruistically. Choice for all—donors, recipients, and physicians—would be enhanced, while lives would be saved.

Interest Groups. Traditionally, Congress has looked to the National Kidney Foundation (NKF) for guidance on matters pertaining to renal disease. The foundation lists as its three major goals the prevention of kidney and urinary tract diseases, the improvement of the well-being of those affected by such diseases, and an increase in the availability of all organs for transplantation.[13]

Despite its stated commitment to increasing the pool of organs, the NKF has assumed a shrill and scolding voice in opposition to incentives of any kind. In 1991, however, the foundation supported pilot trials of incentives for deceased donation. As its leadership has changed over the years, the foundation has closed itself off to new ideas, even with the dearth of kidneys growing far more desperate. It has even sought to stifle discussion. When the American Enterprise Institute held a conference on donor compensation in June 2006, John Davis, the CEO of the foundation, wrote to the president of the institute to say, "We don't see how an AEI forum would contribute substantively to the debate."[14]

The National Kidney Foundation has been a barrier to reform. In 2003 it lobbied strenuously against the James Greenwood and Bill Frist initiatives, both of which outlined incentive plans for deceased donation.[15] According to its policy director, the foundation's National Family Donor Council insists that compensating donors would "cheapen the gift."[16] Whether the council's resistance represents the attitudes of a mere handful of strong-willed members or reflects a large consensus is hard to gauge. In any event, one is compelled to wonder: Does the foundation truly believe that the generous souls who have given their kidneys would deny innocent people a chance to live because other would-be donors don't share their philosophy of giving?

Unfortunately, in 2003, there was no comparable organizational counterweight to the NKF on the matter of donor compensation. An obvious candidate would be the American Association of Kidney Patients (AAKP). In 2004, the AAKP endorsed pilot trials of incentives for deceased donation, but it is reticent about lobbying for the proposal.[17] Similarly, the American Society of Transplant Surgeons (ASTS), the American Society of Transplantation (AST), and the American Medical Association (AMA) have been subdued in their support. The ASTS gingerly endorsed the study of a funeral benefit in 2003 but has since taken no official stand on the virtues of testing incentives.[18] The AMA surely deserves credit for its unflinching testimony endorsing the Greenwood bill at the 2003 hearing—as does UNOS for publicly supporting the AMA and the Association of Organ Procurement Organizations in a call for pilot trials—but all have been passive since.[19] In June 2008, the American Medical Association put financial incentives for deceased donation on its legislative agenda; whether it actively lobbies for pilot trials remains to be seen.[20]

Finally, grassroots activity in favor of incentives is negligible. This inertia may partly reflect the fact that patients with end-stage disease typically feel too physically depleted to take action. Meanwhile, those with greater wherewithal and resources actively seek out donors among their families and friends (who are similarly well endowed with social capital), list themselves with UNOS in multiple regions throughout the country, or even travel overseas. Most likely, the demographics of the afflicted population (whose ranks are dominated by low-income and modestly educated people) in large part account for the failure to organize and advocate for change. Unlike the gay men and middle-class women who have fought, respectively, for treatment and research advances in HIV/AIDS and breast cancer, patients with end-stage renal failure have not managed to attain influence as a group.

Politics. Theoretically, the organ donor compensation debate should not fall along traditional liberal or conservative lines. From a pro-life perspective, for example, concerns about the challenge to human dignity and the specter of bodily commodification are outweighed, in our opinion, by the duty to protect and preserve life. And from a traditionally left-of-center viewpoint, concerns about exploitation of vulnerable individuals, profiteering, and privileging the wealthy could be neutralized by a carefully crafted and tightly monitored compensation system.

Only four Congress members have ever submitted bills or draft bills containing pilot initiatives. None made it out of its respective committee. All were introduced by Republicans. The most recent bill, the 2003 initiative from Representative Greenwood, garnered Democratic support, however; and it is important to remember that Representative Al Gore Jr., a Democrat, raised the possibility of incentives when he introduced NOTA in July 1983.[21] It is an irony of the legislative process that Gore added the prohibition of compensation to NOTA not because of a deeply held belief that incentives were wrong, but because of the unhappy coincidence of his committee's hearings on the bill with the sensational negative publicity attending the startup of an organ brokerage firm in Virginia. But for that one twist of fate, the middle ground between outright prohibition and unregulated markets would most likely have been sown with organ donor compensation programs, and tens of thousands of lives might have been saved in the last quarter-century by an adequate supply of organs generated by appropriate financial incentives.[22]

Among libertarians, compensation systems will inevitably find support because they favor, as a matter of principle, both the application of market approaches and the rights of individuals to do as they wish with their bodies. Libertarians are not a major political force in this country, however.

Proponents of compensated donation recognize—often with keen regret—that altruistic policy is inadequate. Insofar as new laws create new opportunities for individuals to benefit materially from giving a kidney, their virtue lies not in donor enrichment per se or in advancing an ideological point of view, but in the pragmatic attempt to reduce suffering while taking steps to limit unintended consequences.

Just as this book was going to press, a draft bill written by Senator Arlen Specter (R-PA) began circulating in the Senate.[23] The Organ Donor Clarification and Anti-Trafficking Act of 2008 would remove obstacles to rewarding donors while increasing existing penalties on private compensated exchanges, commercial transactions, and brokered sales. The title of the bill reflects Senator Specter's conviction that NOTA never intended to criminalize in-kind incentives provided by state or federal governments to donors or their families. Instead, it was intended to ban commercialization, brokering, and direct monetary exchange.[24] The Specter proposal enables governments to reward those who have donated, thereby encouraging others to do so as well. By opening the door for states to conduct their own pilot projects, this initiative realizes a broader vision than previous incentive bills. The AAKP and AST issued letters of support for the Specter bill and the American Medical Association and American Society of Transplant Surgeons officially endorsed it. This is an encouraging sign that professional and grassroots support for NOTA revision is growing.[25]

There is no denying the political and practical challenges that come with introducing compensation into a quarter-century-old organ procurement scheme built on the premise that generosity is the only legitimate motive for giving. Altruism is, indeed, a most beautiful virtue, yet as death and suffering mount, the construction of an incentive-based program to increase the supply of transplantable human organs—and to suppress unauthorized markets for human organs overseas—has become a moral imperative. Its architects must give serious consideration to principled reservations and to concerns about donor safety, but repugnance and anxiety are not in themselves arguments against innovation. They are only reasons for vigilance.

Appendix A

Organ Transplantation in the United States: A Brief Legislative History

Chad A. Thompson

On December 23, 1954, the first successful kidney transplant from a living donor was performed by Dr. Joseph Murray at Brigham and Women's Hospital, Boston. This breakthrough quickly led to many more kidney transplants, as well as attempts to transplant other organs. The first successful deceased-donor lung transplant took place in 1963, and on December 3, 1967, in Cape Town, South Africa, Christiaan Barnard performed the first successful transplant of a human heart. A few months later, the National Conference of Commissioners on Uniform State Laws (NCCUSL) produced a framework for uniform laws regarding organ and tissue donations across states, since to that point there was no federal law addressing them.

This appendix offers brief summaries of this Uniform Anatomical Gift Act (UAGA) and the principal legislative and policy measures that followed in the subsequent four decades, along with a review of measures that have failed. Of particular interest are two congressional hearings that set out the positions of those who have supported and opposed legislative measures concerning financial incentives for organ donations. These hearings will be examined in some detail at the end.

Major Laws, Passed and Pending

The following are the major laws that have been passed pertaining to organ transplantation and, especially, the procurement and distribution of donor organs, and several measures currently under consideration.

1968 Uniform Anatomical Gift Act. The original Uniform Anatomical Gift Act was not really an act; rather, it was a piece of model legislation drafted by the National Conference of Commissioners on Uniform State Laws on which states could base their own statutes. The purpose was to reduce the differences in states' laws on organ and tissue donation, which to this point had not been handled at the federal level, and to increase the number of available organs by making it easier for people to become organ donors. All fifty states and the District of Columbia adopted the UAGA by 1971.[1] According to the NCCUSL, the 1968 UAGA stipulated for the first time

> that an individual, upon death, could irrevocably donate his or her organs for medical purposes by signing a simple document before witnesses . . . a radical departure from centuries of common-law precedent, which held that a body immediately after death became the property of the next-of-kin.[2]

The UAGA suggested simple forms, such as organ donor cards, for asserting one's wish to be an organ donor, and defined the priority list of those who might donate on behalf of the deceased. Although the first UAGA applied only to organs donated after death and did not explicitly address human organ sales, the use of the word "gift" in the statute's title was commonly interpreted as a barrier to incentives for living donation (although this point has been a matter of some contention). Furthermore, according to Robyn S. Shapiro,

> [While] the original version of UAGA failed to mention commerce in organs explicitly . . . in adopting the 1968 version of UAGA, some states incorporated modifications that do explicitly prohibit organ sales.[3]

1972 Social Security Amendments. In the years following the NCCUSL's drafting and the states' unanimous adoption of the UAGA, continued growth in the numbers of kidney patients, physicians, and treatment centers helped prompt support for federal funding for the treatment of patients with end-stage renal disease (ESRD). In a report to the U.S. Senate Committee on Finance, Senator Vance Hartke wrote,

> In what must be the most tragic irony of the twentieth century, people are dying because they cannot get access to proper medical care. . . . More than 8,000 Americans will die this year from kidney disease who could have been saved if they had been able to afford an artificial kidney machine or transplantation.[4]

Such sentiments prompted the inclusion in the Social Security Amendments of 1972 of a provision extending Medicare coverage for dialysis and kidney transplants to most persons under age sixty-five suffering from chronic kidney disease.[5] The legislation, in turn, significantly increased the demand for kidney transplants, with yearly expenditures in the Medicare ESRD program growing from $5.4 billion in 1991 to over $18.3 billion in 2004.[6]

1984 National Organ Transplant Act. According to Kant Patel and Mark Rushefsky, the approval of cyclosporine for commercial use in 1983 was "one of the most important developments in the history of organ transplants."[7] The appearance of this "revolutionary antirejection drug" sparked a huge increase in transplants and a survival success rate that soon drove the demand for organs well beyond the supply and made imperative the implementation of a system of equitable distribution. The lack of a national mechanism that could manage and fairly allocate scarce organs would lead to the passage in October 1984 of the National Organ Transplant Act (NOTA), the first federal legislation designed to regulate organ transplants.

NOTA was the product of eleven congressional hearings and extensive debate. The specific catalyst for legislative action was not the shortage of kidneys, but rather the impact of cyclosporine on the demand for liver transplants.[8] People desperate for suitable organs and/or lacking the funds to secure places on the waiting list mounted media campaigns and organized countless fundraisers. Politicians were bombarded with pleas for help. President Ronald Reagan even made organ transplantation the focal point of his weekly radio address on at least one occasion, offering to provide Air Force jet and helicopter transportation if donors could be found for a few select transplant candidates.[9] The furor surrounding liver transplants prompted Donald Denny, then director of organ procurement for the Transplant Foundation at the University of Pittsburgh, to point out at a congressional hearing that

> the shortage of kidneys for transplantation has received relatively little attention, largely because renal transplantation is not a form of transplant therapy which is often an alternative to death. . . . The undeniable facts that a real kidney, a transplanted kidney, provides a better quality of life for ESRD patients and that renal transplantation is more cost-effective per patient life-year than the artificial kidney have not been sufficient to cause the national sense of urgency which underlies these hearings. Without intending to diminish the meaning and the importance of this sub-committee's purpose today, I must lament . . . the fact that recent publicity concerning the need for liver transplants for a handful of patients at two or three transplant centers (including my own) has outweighed the silent suffering of many thousands of patients waiting for a kidney transplant at 150 transplant hospitals over the past decade in moving the conscience of this nation.[10]

Initial testimonies during the NOTA hearings focused on improving the coordination of organ retrieval and the effectiveness of organ procurement organizations. These early hearings held little opposition to incentives for organ donation. Representative Al Gore Jr. of Tennessee, who championed NOTA and hosted many of the hearings, felt that incentives would be necessary if there proved to be a shortage of altruistic organ donations.[11] According to Jerold R. Mande, later a health policy advisor to the White House, who worked for Gore at the time and helped organize the NOTA hearings,

> Gore objected to a marketplace for organs for moral/ethical reasons well before the [Jacobs] hearing. Nevertheless, he ordered

an investigation that considered seriously any idea that could alleviate the tragic shortage of organs. He waited until we completed our investigation before taking a public stand. We considered all systems that might increase organ/donor supply including the use of various incentives. We spoke to many respectable advocates of the use of markets. After concluding markets were more likely to hurt than help organ/donor supply, we organized a hearing scripted to make that point.[12]

Fears that organ brokering and private market exchanges would decrease the supply of transplantable organs, harm the quality of the organs, and exploit the poor eventually led to the inclusion in NOTA of section 301, entitled "Prohibition of Organ Purchases." The section imposes criminal penalties of up to $50,000 and five years in prison on any person who "knowingly acquire[s], receive[s], or otherwise transfer[s] any human organ for valuable consideration for use in human transplantation if the transfer affects interstate commerce."[13] Not included in the definition of "valuable consideration," according to the act, were "reasonable payments associated with the removal, transportation, implantation, processing, preservation, quality control, and storage of a human organ or the expenses of travel, housing, and lost wages incurred by the donor of a human organ in connection with the donation of the organ."[14]

Beyond this, however, what constituted "valuable consideration" was unclear, and the question would become key to future legislative debates on organ transplantation. According to the Congressional Research Service (CRS), "The legislative history of the 1984 NOTA does not discuss the meaning of the term. . . . It simply expresses Congress's intent to criminalize the buying and selling of organs for profit."[15] The CRS report goes on:

The House conference report for [S. 2048] reiterated that Section 301 was directed toward monetary exchanges: "This title intends to make the buying and selling of human organs unlawful. . . . " During congressional hearings in 2003 on incentives to increase organ donations, strong objections were proffered against the use of direct monetary incentives to procure organs.[16]

Most of the people involved in the NOTA hearings were adamantly opposed to incentives, and although three witnesses spoke out against the ban on them,[17] they were unable to sway lawmakers. NOTA received little opposition in the House or Senate.[18]

Under NOTA, the U.S. Department of Health and Human Services established the nonprofit Organ Procurement and Transplantation Network (OPTN), whose mission was, among other directives, to "conduct and participate in systematic efforts . . . to acquire all useable organs from potential donors" and "to have a system to allocate donated organs equitably among transplant patients according to established medical criteria."[19] In 1986, a contract to operate the OPTN was awarded to the United Network for Organ Sharing.

Finally, the 1984 NOTA established a twenty-five–member Task Force on Organ Transplantation to study and advise on transplant policy issues, including the procurement and distribution of donor organs.

1986 Omnibus Budget Reconciliation Act. The Omnibus Budget Reconciliation Act of 1986 superseded state laws whose aim, according to Kathleen Andersen and Daniel Fox, was "to increase the potential donor pool by requiring hospital personnel to request consent of potential candidates or their families for donation, or at least inform people of the option."[20] The act mandated that all hospitals participating in Medicare or Medicaid develop procedures to establish

> protocols for organ procurement and standards for organ procurement agencies [including] written protocols for the identification of potential organ donors that—
>
> (i) assure that families of potential organ donors are made aware of the option of organ or tissue donation and their option to decline,
>
> (ii) encourage discretion and sensitivity with respect to the circumstances, views, and beliefs of such families, and

(iii) require that such hospital's designated organ procurement agency . . . is notified of potential organ donors.[21]

Each hospital that performed organ transplants was also required to be a
member of, and abide by the rules and requirements of, the OPTN.[22]

This legislation was significant because it required hospitals to develop
programs designed to increase organ donation, or risk losing a vital source
of government funding.

1987 Uniform Anatomical Gift Act. In 1987 the NCCUSL updated the
Uniform Anatomical Gift Act[23] to address issues that had arisen in organ
transplantation since the drafting of the 1968 UAGA and to attempt to remedy the failure of current policy to "produce a sufficient supply of organs to
meet the current or projected demand for them."[24] The revised UAGA
guaranteed priority of a decedent's wishes over those of the decedent's
family members; streamlined the process of completing the necessary doc-
uments to effect organ donation; mandated that hospitals and emergency
personnel develop procedures of routine inquiry and required request—
that is, protocols for asking patients upon admission to the hospital (or
their families, if the patients died), if they were to be organ donors; and permitted medical examiners and coroners to provide transplantable organs
from subjects of autopsies and investigations under certain conditions.[25]
Most notably, where the 1968 UAGA did not address the commercial sale
and purchase of human organs, the 1987 version followed NOTA in explicitly prohibiting them, although the UAGA specified that the ban pertained
to body parts whose removal was "intended to occur after the death of
the decedent." The NCCUSL committee that prepared the act commented
that this section did "not cover the sale by living donors if removal [was]
intended to occur before death."[26]

While the 1968 UAGA enjoyed unanimous approval by all fifty states
and the District of Columbia, the 1987 UAGA was opposed by many states
and adopted in only twenty-six.[27] Debate did not involve the ban on organ
sales but focused rather on the priority of donor's intent over family objections, required request language, and language that could allow medical
examiners to donate a deceased individual's organs or other body parts.[28]
Although it was intended to create uniformity among the various state

statutes that had been passed to fill gaps left by the 1968 act, several states enacted transplant legislation on their own rather than ratify the 1987 UAGA legislation.[29]

1991 Patient Self-Determination Act. The federal Patient Self-Determination Act (PSDA)[30] was adopted in 1991 to encourage the use of advance directives, such as living wills and durable powers of attorney for health care,[31] and to reinforce the idea of patient autonomy. The legislation was intended to ensure doctors' awareness of, and compliance with, patients' instructions for care in terminal phases of their illnesses, including the use of organs for transplantation.

1999 Organ Donor Leave Act. The Organ Donor Leave Act, signed by President Bill Clinton and passed in September 1999, provided a federal employee with seven days of paid leave in any calendar year to be a bone marrow donor and thirty days of paid leave to be an organ donor.[32]

2004 Organ Donation and Recovery Improvement Act. The Organ Donation and Recovery Improvement Act was, the Congressional Research Service reports, "the first federal law directly applicable in part to living donors."[33] Introduced by Senator Bill Frist of Tennessee as S. 573 and by Representative Michael Bilirakas of Florida as H.R. 399,[34] both bills included sections calling for demonstration projects to increase organ donation. The Frist bill required the U.S. Department of Health and Human Services to provide a report evaluating the ethical implications of proposals for demonstration projects to increase donation of organs from cadavers, and stated that "notwithstanding section 301 of the National Organ Transplant Act (42 USC 274e), upon the submission of and consistent with the report by the Secretary . . . the Secretary may conduct up to 3 demonstration projects to increase cadaveric donation."[35]

This language might eventually have opened the door to demonstration projects for financial incentives, but it was not included in the final version of the bill, which became the Organ Donation and Recovery Improvement Act and was enacted in April 2004.[36] The language was allegedly removed in response to efforts by Dr. Francis Delmonico of the National Kidney Foundation.[37] The bill did seek to reduce financial disincentives for living donors by reimbursing travel and subsistence expenses for low-income donors, and this portion was included in the law. It never received Appropriations Committee funding. In 2007 the Health Resources and Services Administration and the Division of Transplantation, both within the Department of Health and Human Services, initiated a four-year grant program to reimburse donors who qualify as having financial hardship. Funding is provided by HHS. Reimbursement cannot exceed $6,000.[38]

2006 Uniform Anatomical Gift Act. In July 2006, the NCCUSL approved yet another new version of the UAGA that comported with changes in federal law providing for an organ allocation system through hospitals and procurement organizations. The new UAGA expanded the list of persons who could make an anatomical gift on behalf of the deceased in the event that no determination had been made prior to death, and it bolstered the rule that a donor's decision to make an anatomical gift was not subject to change by others.[39] The updated UAGA has been approved by the American Bar Association and endorsed by the American Medical Association, the American Academy of Ophthalmology, the American Association of Tissue Banks, the American Society of Cataract and Refractive Surgery, the Association of Organ Procurement Organizations, the Cornea Society, the Eye Bank Association of America, the National Kidney Foundation, and the United Network for Organ Sharing.[40] As of November 2008, it had been enacted by thirty-four states and the District of Columbia.[41]

2007 Charlie W. Norwood Living Organ Donation Act. Two new medical options for living kidney donation have recently been introduced, and legislation has already been passed to address issues raised by one of these innovations. In a March 8, 2007, report for Congress, the Congressional Research Service explains that in paired and list donation,

> willing living donors who are [biologically] incompatible with their intended recipients agree to donate their organs to an unknown recipient. In exchange, their intended recipient either receives an organ (paired donation), or a higher spot on the waiting list (list donation).[42]

The Charlie W. Norwood Living Organ Donation Act received unanimous approval in both the House and Senate, and was signed into law by President Bush on December 21, 2007. This law amended the National Organ Transplant Act to clarify that kidney paired donation did not involve the transfer of a human organ for valuable consideration.[43] (A previous version, S. 2306, that was introduced in the previous Congress, also included list donation.) Representative Norwood's office reported that a preliminary analysis by the Congressional Budget Office estimated the bill would realize savings of $30 million over five years, and $500 million over ten. An official Congressional Budget Office estimate does not exist.[44]

2007 Living Donor Job Security Act. Proposed in three previous sessions of Congress, the Living Donor Job Security Act is currently in committee. H.R. 2808 was introduced by Representative Rubén Hinojosa of Texas and has twelve cosponsors. It would amend the Family and Medical Leave Act of 1993 (FMLA) to entitle employees to unpaid leave from their jobs to provide living organ donations. Employers covered by FMLA include "public service employers, all primary and secondary schools, and all employers who have fifty or more employees for at least twenty of the calendar work weeks."[45]

2008 Stephanie Tubbs-Jones Gift of Life Medal Act. Establishes the Stephanie Tubbs-Jones Gift of Life Medal for organ donors and the families of organ donors. The act was signed by President Bush in October 2008, weeks after the sudden death of Tubbs-Jones, who was an organ donor. She was a congresswoman from Ohio.

Other Efforts by the States. Many states have made efforts to reduce disincentives and/or to provide mild incentives to encourage organ donations. At least eleven states allow $10,000 tax deductions for travel, lodging, and lost wages that are not reimbursed.[46] At least twenty-nine provide varying amounts of paid or unpaid leave from work for bone marrow and/or organ donors.[47] At least eight states require that companies allow a leave of absence for private-sector employees who donate.[48] During his years as governor of Wisconsin, former secretary of health and human services Tommy Thompson implemented programs to encourage donation, such as holding an annual ceremony and awarding a Governor's Medal to honor donors and their families.[49] Kentucky, Maine, and New York each dedicate a day or a week to recognizing donors.

Other states have contemplated innovative and sometimes controversial programs to increase donations. South Carolina discussed shortening prison sentences for inmates who decide to donate organs.[50] Georgia provided driver's license discounts to anyone who signed up to be an organ donor until July 2005, when the program was discontinued.[51] A 1994 Pennsylvania plan would have provided $300 toward funeral expenses for anyone in the state whose organs were donated after death, but it was never implemented.[52]

Failed Federal Proposals

The following are brief descriptions of proposed legislation concerning financial incentives for organ donation that did not become law. They are notable in illustrating the various means with which policymakers have experimented, unsuccessfully, in the past few decades to compensate organ donors (or their families) for their "gift of life."

Crane Bill. On June 3, 1981, Representative Philip Crane of Illinois introduced a bill that would have offered tax incentives for transplantable organs from deceased donors. H.R. 3774 proposed "a $25,000 deduction on the [donor's] last taxable year plus a $25,000 exclusion from estate taxes," with the same incentives going to the family of a child donor.[53] It was referred to the House Ways and Means Subcommittee on Health on February 16, 1982 and died in committee. The same bill, under the designation H.R. 540, was brought up again during the 98th Congress by Rep. Philip Crane of Illinois on January 6, 1983. It was again referred to the Ways and Means Subcommittee on Health on January 14, 1983, where it again died in committee. A similar bill was introduced again on January 3, 1989 by Rep. Joseph Kolter of Pennsylvania as H.R. 242 in the 101st Congress ("Transplant Assistance Act of 1989"). The last major action on this bill was a referral to Energy and Commerce's Subcommittee on Health and the Environment (though House Ways and Means is recorded to have had its hands on it for some time before this final referral) on February 6, 1989.[54]

Greenwood Bills. In November 1999, Representative James Greenwood of Pennsylvania introduced H.R. 3471 "to authorize the Secretary of Health and Human Services to carry out demonstration projects to increase the supply of organs donated for human transplantation." The bill would have allowed projects to establish financial incentives for organ donation, including the payment of travel and subsistence expenses incurred by individuals making live donations, and it would have required that one or more of these projects provide payments for the purchase of life insurance policies or annuities, payable to a donor's designee.[55] The bill had no cosponsors and abruptly died in committee.

Representative Greenwood subsequently introduced similar bills, H.R. 5224 in July 2002 and H.R. 2856 in July 2003. Both bills had five cosponsors—a small improvement over H.R. 3471—but after their introduction no action was taken by the committee.[56]

Gift of Life Congressional Medal Act. On a number of occasions, Senator Bill Frist and others have proposed national medals to be given to organ donors and/or their families. The bills generally have had several cosponsors, but they have never made it out of committee.[57]

Living Organ Donation Incentives Act. Proposed by Representative Karen Thurman of Florida in 1999, the Living Organ Donation Incentives Act, like the more recent Living Donor Job Security Act (see above) sought to amend the Family and Medical Leave Act of 1993 to allow unpaid leave for individuals to be organ donors, as well as amend the 1946 Public Health Service Act to provide funding for travel and other expenses related to organ donation. The bill, which would also have increased the federal payment rate for renal dialysis services by 2.9 percent, had thirty-four cosponsors and received attention in several committees, but no further action was taken.[58]

Gift of Life Tax Credit Act. In 2000 and 2001, Representative James Hansen of Utah introduced the Gift of Life Tax Credit Act, which would have amended the Internal Revenue Code to allow a (refundable) $10,000 credit to individuals who donated their organs at death.[59] When the bill was proposed in 2000 it had twenty-two cosponsors, but only five in 2001. Both times it was immediately referred to the

House Committee on Ways and Means, and no further action was taken.[60]

Help Organ Procurement Expand Act. In 2000 and 2001, Representative Christopher Smith of New Jersey introduced the Help Organ Procurement Expand Act, which would have provided a $2,500 tax credit to individuals who donated their organs while living, or to the designated beneficiaries or estates of individuals who donated their organs after death. The bill was referred to the House Committee on Ways and Means, and no further action was taken.[61]

Living Organ Donor Tax Credit Act. In 2005 and again in 2007, Representative Joe Wilson of South Carolina introduced the Living Organ Donor Tax Credit Act, which would have allowed a nonrefundable tax credit for any unreimbursed costs or lost wages, up to $5,000, associated with a living organ donation. It would have provided for this by amending the Public Health Service Act to exclude such a tax credit from being considered as valuable consideration for the donation. The bill was referred to the Subcommittee on Health, of the House Committee on Energy and Commerce. No further action was taken.[62]

Congressional Hearings

In terms of legislative history, the question of providing financial incentives to living organ donors has so far not even emerged as an issue. To date, practically the only formal discussion by lawmakers with reference to living donors has concerned the elimination of disincentives—for instance, by compensating donors for lost wages or travel expenses related to the surgery—which has not been much of an argument at all. Any real debates involving incentives have pertained strictly to deceased donors.[63]

While some of the ethical concerns are the same for deceased and living donors (such as worries about the "commodification" of human organs), differences between the two cases are considerable, and it is not terribly helpful here to review the literature regarding views toward living-donor incentives when they are not in legislative play. Still, we can gain insights and draw inferences about the legalization of financial incentives for living organ donors from advocates' positions for and against deceased-donor incentives. Perhaps the most expedient way to do so is to examine briefly testimony given in two congressional hearings that were held on the subject of increasing the supply of donor organs, on April 15, 1999, and June 3, 2003, respectively. While neither resulted in any legislation, the hearings provided venues for representatives of groups that have been at the forefront of the incentives debate to make clear where their organizations stood.

Putting Patients First: Increasing Organ Supply for Transplantation. In 1999, the House of Representatives' Subcommittee on Health and Environment, of the Committee on Commerce, held a hearing entitled, *Putting Patients First: Increasing Organ Supply for Transplantation.* Representative James Greenwood of Pennsylvania proposed a federally funded, $10,000 life insurance policy for everyone in the United States, with benefits payable upon donation and transplantation of the deceased's organs. One of Greenwood's constituents brought a check for $100,000 to help start the program. Pennsylvania's plan to provide $300 toward funeral expenses for donors also figured prominently in the discussion.[64] Represented at the hearing were, among others, the American Society of Transplantation, the American Society of Transplant Surgeons, the LifeLink Foundation (which operates the organ procurement program for the state of Florida), and the National Kidney Foundation, along with a number of transplant programs from different parts of the United States. The focus was on initiating programs—such as the life insurance benefit—to increase the number of Americans willing to pledge their organs for transplantation at the time of their deaths, and to encourage and educate families to follow through on these choices.

Witnesses at the hearing were fairly unanimous in their approval of these proposed deceased-donor incentive programs, particularly if they might serve as pilot studies for broader initiatives. According to spokesman John F. Neylan, the American Society of Transplantation would be in favor of "carrying out creative pilot studies to explore the possibility that quite modest financial supports may enhance organ donation," such as that offered by the Pennsylvania program. "We need to be open," Neylan said, "even to the idea of financial incentives, but it needs to be done carefully."[65]

Joshua Miller, president of the American Society of Transplant Surgeons, also commenting on the Pennsylvania program, suggested that "if you would have asked this question 25 years ago . . . it would have been an absolute no . . . but I think you have got to look at this again and again and again. . . . I personally see no ethical issue."[66]

John R. Campbell, executive director of the LifeLink Foundation, was somewhat more cautious. "We believe this will provide the organ donation and transplantation community an opportunity to view Pennsylvania as a pilot state for the rest of the nation. . . . If rates of donation increase, we may want to consider a similar initiative," Campbell stated. "However," he added,

> we are concerned about the possibility that any incentive system will be viewed by potential donor families as inappropriate when these families consider giving the priceless gift of life. We believe other programs, such as LifeLink's, have been shown to be effective without stipends.[67]

The most negative response to incentives proposals at the 1999 hearing came from Robert S. D. Higgins, director of thoracic organ transplantation at Henry Ford Hospital in Detroit, Michigan. "We question the advisability," he testified, "of tying financial incentives to a system which has been based upon altruism and voluntary donations of organs." He continued,

> The "who", "how", and "why" of donating organs [from deceased individuals] are unclear to many, and adding a new dimension with monetary incentives may cloud or create even more suspicion during the sensitive decision making period by family members. The potential for coercive economic incentives that may undercut the altruistic nature of donation and create questionable motivation for donation, in particular for those who are in financial need, is a significant concern. . . . Even small amounts begin the danger of starting down a slippery slope that can lead to the dangers of a payment system for organs.

Even so, Higgins acknowledged that

clearly defined financial incentives such [as] "rewarded gifting" in the form of modest sums of money paid to a family to defray costs of funeral expenses may benefit individual transplant recipients and the society at large. These kinds of initiatives, of course, would have to be carefully delineated, so as not to be construed as a payment system for organs.[68]

One of the most positive responses came from Joseph L. Brand, chairman of the Office of Scientific and Public Policy at the National Kidney Foundation. "We have looked at this issue with our constituents," Brand stated, "and the bottom line is, we would support at least a pilot study on financial incentives." He went on:

> Financial incentives, if we have any data that says they are working, we ought to try them elsewhere. So we certainly would support that. . . . The National Kidney Foundation has long called for demonstration projects to determine the impact of programs which would assist donor families in paying for funeral or burial expenses.[69]

Assessing Initiatives to Increase Organ Donations. In 2003, another congressional hearing was held to discuss strategies to increase the organ supply. *Assessing Initiatives to Increase Organ Donations* was conducted before the House's Subcommittee of Oversight and Investigations, of the Committee on Energy and Commerce. Once again, representatives of a number of organizations at the forefront of organ transplantation set forth their respective positions on financial incentives for deceased-donor organ donations.

Perhaps aware that the eventuality of incentives for living donors was not quite as remote as it had been in 1999, some speakers were a bit more reserved in their expressions of support for any legislative efforts to change the long-standing NOTA policy prohibiting "valuable consideration" for organ donations than their colleagues had been at that earlier hearing. Robert M. Sade, a professor of surgery at Medical University of South Carolina and a member of the American Medical Association's Council on Ethical and Judicial Affairs, said the AMA encouraged "the medical community to support the reexamination of motivation for cadaveric organ donation," but he was careful to specify that "the studies should be limited to understanding motivation for cadaveric organ donation only, and not its effect on living donors."[70]

Joseph Roth, president-elect of the Association of Organ Procurement Organizations, stated that the AOPO would support pilot projects for incentives whose "shape" was "determined by the entire community and not just by AOPO";[71] Robert Metzger, president-elect of the United Network for Organ Sharing (UNOS), said his organization "in essence . . . backed the AMA stance."[72] Neither, however, mentioned incentives in his prepared statement, having concentrated instead mainly on advocating educational and public relations initiatives and organizational efforts within the transplant community; they brought up their views on incentives only when prompted by Greenwood.

Abraham Shaked, president of the American Society of Transplant Surgeons, declared his organization's continuing interest in studying "various methods and programs to increase donation rates that may have a financial component," such as offering "a modest funeral expense benefit to the family of a decedent donor, not as a payment for a donated organ, but as a token of thanks," and reiterated the ASTS's support for "initiatives to eliminate financial disincentives to donation."[73] Shaked was much more plainspoken, however, than his predecessor Joshua Miller had been in 1999 in expressing the organization's strong opposition "to the buying, selling, or brokering of organs for transplantation in agreement with the National Organ Transplant Act (NOTA) which makes it illegal to exchange organs for 'valuable consideration.'"[74] Such activity would run the risk of turning a "gift of life" into a commodity to be bought and sold—a signal to the international "black market" that the United States tolerates the commodification of human organs.[75]

Furthest toward the negative side of the debate was the National Kidney Foundation, whose position also stood in contrast to the enthusiasm its representative had expressed for demonstration projects four years earlier. While Representative Greenwood, chairman of the subcommittee, declared that "saving an additional life or thousands of lives certainly overcomes any ethical argument" against creating a financial incentive, NFK spokesman Francis L. Delmonico was most emphatic in his opposition to offering such incentives for organ donation—even from deceased donors:

> Any attempt to assign a monetary value to the human body or its body parts, even in the hope of increasing organ supply, diminishes human dignity and devaluates the very human life we seek to save. Proponents of financial incentives for non-living organ donation assert that demonstration projects should be conducted to determine whether it will increase the organ supply. However, the NKF believes that it is impossible to separate the ethical debate of financial incentives for non-living donation from the unethical practice of selling human organs.[76]

Delmonico spoke of awful headlines that would result from congressional endorsement of financial incentives, claimed that allowing incentives would corrupt the doctor/patient relationship, and argued that the integrity of the donor pool would be harmed.[77] Responding to Delmonico, Greenwood offered the most direct statement on incentives to living organ donors uttered in either hearing:

> You had indicated . . . something to the effect that it would be impossible to distinguish between financial incentives that went to a decedent's estate versus buying an organ from a living person and creating that incentive. And I want to challenge that assertion, because I think people don't have a lot of difficulty making discrimination between someone who is alive and someone who is dead. And, obviously, since no one that I am aware of is advocating a policy that would actually pay someone to donate a kidney while they are alive, I think that is ethically abhorrent to all of us. You are putting that person's life at risk.[78]

In the light of this argument from one of the strongest proponents of organ-donor incentives, any serious legislative consideration of financial incentives for living donors, beyond compensation for donation-related expenses, would appear to have remained a long way off.

Appendix B

Evolution of an Idea

Sally Satel

The use of monetary incentives as motivation for people to give up kidneys is not at all a new idea; it has been around for nearly four decades. The following chronology lists important milestones in the public's growing awareness of the organ shortage, and in developing attitudes toward donor compensation as a means to address it.

1966. Thirteen years after the first successful kidney transplant has taken place, the Ciba Foundation of London sponsors what might be the first conference on the ethics of transplantation. "Since it is ethically acceptable to sell blood," asks one prescient participant, "is it also ethically acceptable to sell major organs? This may not be a pressing issue now but it probably will be so in five or ten years' time."[1]

1970. The supply of organs for transplantation is already insufficient, according to eminent transplant surgeon Thomas E. Starzl of the University of Pittsburgh.[2] The first of a handful of scholarly articles that will be published in the 1970s appears, suggesting a role for markets or in-kind transactions for both live and cadaver kidneys. Notably, these articles are produced by legal scholars and economists, not physicians. "Swift advances in organ transplantation are forcing us to think about what was once unthinkable: buying human organs," writes a UCLA law professor.[3]

1977. An economist presents a particularly detailed discussion of what kinds of incentives might be offered, and an apparatus for making them available.[4]

149

1983. With the introduction in the early 1980s of cyclosporine, a break-through immunosuppressant medication, transplants have become more successful, and the demand for donor organs has begun to soar.[5] In one of the earliest appearances of the incentives issue in the news media, the author of a *Wall Street Journal* opinion article entitled "Providing Incentives for Organ Donations" writes, "Some people think that any intrusion of money into medical matters is morally wrong, [but] in the new age created by the availability of cyclosporine, a more realistic and pragmatic attitude is required."[6]

1984. The creation of the United Network for Organ Sharing (UNOS) registry by the National Organ Transplant Act (NOTA) reflects the progress being made in the field of organ transplantation.

1985. The *Washington Post* describes a group called the Transplant Society, which plans to enroll individuals ("members") who are interested in having $10,000 donated to charity in their names if they agree to have their organs harvested at death, and if the organs are successfully retrieved. Upon enrolling, these members and their families will become priority recipients for organs donated through the Transplant Society. The international Transplantation Society explicitly states that payments are ethically allowable.[7] Around this same time, detailed proposals for futures markets in organs, wherein individuals sign contracts to sell their organs at death, begin to appear.[8]

1988. In June, a symposium at Vanderbilt University gathers leaders in a wide variety of fields to synthesize the current state of knowledge concerning organ transplantation policy, including the possibility of payment for organs.[9]

1991. Transplant surgeon Thomas Peters becomes the first physician to call for compensation for families of deceased organ donors in a major medical journal. In an article published in the *Journal of the American Medical Association*, Peters suggests that a death benefit of $1,000, financed by the federal government, be offered to loved ones.[10] By now, the subject of the organ shortage is sufficiently familiar for a *Time*/CNN poll to ask people what they would do if they "or a close relative had a fatal disease that could possibly be cured by the transplant." Fifty-six percent of respondents say they would "purchase the necessary organ or tissue."[11] A National Kidney

Foundation Consensus Conference called "Controversies in Organ Donation" holds a panel to contemplate incentives. The panel makes two recommendations for demonstration projects: a program in which individuals would declare in advance their interest in having a payment made to their estates at death, and a program in which families would be offered burial expenses.[12] The U.S. surgeon general holds a workshop called "Increasing Organ Donation," and incentives are endorsed by some of the participants.[13]

1992. The *Wall Street Journal* reports on recent developments in the ongoing discussion on donor compensation in an article headlined "Scarcity of Organs for Transplant Sparks a Move to Legalize Financial Incentives." The article quotes a frustrated transplant surgeon from Chicago who asks, "When are we going to stop talking and do something?"[14]

1993. At a congressional hearing on NOTA, the National Kidney Foundation (NKF) proposes in its testimony that the law be changed to permit payments of burial expenses for donors. Its spokesperson suggests that a "standardized and small" amount, perhaps $2,000, be given through an agency, such as the Health Care Financing Administration, to "a third party, like a funeral director."[15] A white paper by UNOS deems incentives for deceased donation "ethically justifiable only if found preferable to the other feasible options to increase donations."[16]

1995. The American Medical Association engages the matter through its Council on Ethical and Judicial Affairs, which concludes that forms of financial incentives that stop short of outright cash payment "may be ethically permissible" and suggests that a pilot study be conducted.[17]

1997. The increased visibility of the issue prompts the writing of "The Bellagio Task Force Report on Transplantation, Bodily Integrity, and the International Traffic in Organs." Sponsored by Columbia University, the task force finds "no unarguable ethical principle that would justify a ban on the sale of organs under all circumstances."[18]

1999. The NKF approves a plan by the state of Pennsylvania to offer a $300 burial benefit to families who donate their loved ones' organs (with the cash going directly to a funeral home). "We are not talking about a situation where the organ goes to the highest bidder, or that there should be market for organs. We are talking about a limited, specified amount of money paid to a third party," the foundation's director of scientific and public policy tells the *New York Times*.[19]

2001. Pleas for reform have been growing more insistent, and the academic literature on incentives has blossomed.[20] Anthropologist Donald Joralemon observes that "a vehement rejection on ethical grounds of anything but uncompensated donation—once the professional norm—has slowly been replaced by an open debate of plans that offer financial rewards to persons willing to have their organs, or the organs of deceased kin, taken for transplantation."[21]

2002. The Advisory Committee on Organ Transplantation of the Department of Health and Human Services recommends a demonstration project on incentives for deceased donations.[22] The American Medical Association's House of Delegates votes to endorse the opinion of its Council on Ethical and Judicial Affairs that the impact of financial incentives on organ donation should be studied.[23] On the global front, the International Congress on the Ethics of Organ Transplantation passes a resolution urging innovation, stating, "Individual countries will need to study alternative, locally relevant models, considered ethical in their societies, which would increase the number of transplants, protect and respect the donor, and reduce the likelihood of rampant, unregulated commerce."[24]

2003. The American Medical Association testifies on behalf of legislation that would permit pilot studies of incentives for deceased-donor organs.[25] UNOS supports the AMA, and the Association of Organ Procurement Organizations also speaks out in favor of the legislation.[26]

2004. The reformer mentality within the transplant establishment is personified by Dr. Hans Sollinger, chairman of the Division of Transplantation at the University of Wisconsin. A member of the Secretary's Advisory Committee on Transplantation (ACOT), Sollinger says, "Two years ago I would have been happy with the current position of not allowing any discussion about buying and selling organs, but not now. Ads in the newspaper, the donor case in Denver, more and more people on dialysis, has me wondering if we shouldn't revisit the question."[27] At the November meeting of ACOT, its Valuable Consideration Subcommittee adopts a proposal recommending that the secretary of health and human services be given regulatory authority to define "valuable consideration."[28]

2005–6. Three academic books on the virtues of organ markets are published.[29]

2006. An address by Dr. Richard Fine, president of the American Society of Transplantation (AST), to the first World Transplant Congress in Boston offers striking evidence of how far the donor compensation debate has evolved: "Is it wrong for an individual, who wishes to utilize part of his body for the benefit of another [to] be provided with financial compensation that could obliterate a life of destitution for the individual and his family?" he asks his colleagues. "It is time that we cease to be pious about 'equity' in the acquisition of solid organs for transplantation."[30]

2007. Jeffrey Crippen of the AST and Arthur Matas of the American Society of Transplant Surgeons (ASTS) support trials of financial incentives in their presidential addresses at the second World Transplant Congress.[31] An informal poll taken at the annual meeting of the ASTS suggests considerable support for Fine's sentiments, revealing that 80 to 85 percent of members are in favor of studying incentives for living donors.[32]

2008. The American Medical Association House of Delegates votes to lobby for legislative changes that would allow pilot studies to find out if offering financial incentives would increase the number of organs available for transplantation from deceased donors. The resolution places financial incentives on the AMA's legislative agenda for the first time.[33]

2008. Senator Arlen Specter (R-PA) is developing the Organ Donor Clarification Act of 2008 (ODCA). The bill redefines valuable consideration to exclude in-kind rewards offered to donors by federal, state, or local governments. Private sales remain illegal and the penalties are increased. The American Association of Kidney Patients, the American Society of Transplantation, and the American Medical Association offer official support of the draft version of ODCA.[34]

Appendix C

Public Attitudes

Sally Satel

Where do Americans stand on the issue of compensation for organs from deceased and living individuals? Overall, polls and surveys have shown the public to be amenable to the idea.[1]

Attitudes toward incentives for organ donation have been explored along two dimensions: attitudes regarding remuneration of donors as a matter of policy, and personal judgments about whether payment would influence respondents' motivation to donate their own organs or those of loved ones. Only one poll—the Time/CNN poll—posed the urgent question of what respondents would actually do if they themselves or a close relative had a fatal disease and needed an organ to be cured. In it, 56 percent of respondents said they would "purchase the necessary organ or tissue."[2]

Incentives as Policy

Polls on incentives have yielded results generally favorable toward allowing them. An exception was one of the earliest—a 1986 government survey—in which a robust majority, 78 percent, rejected the idea that families should be paid for granting permission to retrieve organs. Notably, the survey presented a scenario in which grieving families were offered money at the time of their loved ones' death. This could have been interpreted as insensitive.[3]

Respondents to subsequent inquiries were considerably more receptive. In a joint survey by the United Network for Organ Sharing (UNOS) and the National Kidney Foundation (NKF), published in 1992, 48 percent felt

154

that some form of financial or nonfinancial compensation should be offered to increase the number of deceased-donor organs available, with 42 percent opposed and 10 percent undecided. Among those ages eighteen to twenty-four, 65 percent were in favor.[4] These findings prompted the NKF vice chairman at the time, Alan Hull, MD, to observe that "some states should be convinced to conduct pilot studies" on offering financial incentives.[5] Much more recently, a 2007 poll conducted by Harris Interactive for the *Wall Street Journal* found 49 percent of adults in Harris's online panel sample somewhat or strongly in favor of incentives.[6] Notably, these respondents were assuming a traditional free-market model; a model in which non-cash incentives were offered to the donors and the organs distributed by algorithm would have helped resolve respondents' concerns about privileging the wealthy at the expense of the poor.

Surveys conducted of groups other than nationally representative samples included a 1993 door-to-door survey of 150 Canadians (yielding 100 usable responses). Respondents were given two case vignettes and asked whether the needy individual in each vignette should "be allowed to buy a kidney." Sixty-nine percent answered yes to one vignette and 74 percent to the other.[7] A 1999 poll found only 12 percent of 400 college students offended by the idea of offering incentives for donation at death, suggesting that age may play a meaningful role in attitudes toward donor compensation.[8] A 2005 academic survey of roughly 1,000 Pennsylvania residents reported 59 percent favorable to the general idea of incentives, with 53 percent saying direct payments to families of potential deceased donors would be acceptable.[9] Dialysis patients in a 1997 survey placed a greater emphasis on increasing the supply of kidneys through incentives than maintaining an altruistic system of organ donation.[10]

A 2006 national telephone survey of 845 individuals conducted by a team from the Johns Hopkins School of Public Health examined attitudes toward the acceptability of incentives by race and ethnicity.[11] Among African-American and Hispanic subjects who indicated willingness to become living donors, 50 percent and 70 percent, respectively, endorsed tax breaks, payment from government, or payment by employers to living donors.[12] Finally, a recent poll from the Netherlands reported 62 percent unopposed to a system of procurement based on compensation, although only one-fourth of those said they would personally participate in such a transaction.[13]

Incentives and Personal Decision-Making

Across surveys, most respondents report that incentives would not affect their willingness to donate, but among those who say they would, the net effect was generally to increase motivation, especially among young adults. A nationwide sampling of over 6,000 Americans published in 1997 found that cash or in-kind rewards (unspecified in terms of monetary value) would inspire 12 percent to be more likely to donate their loved ones' organs while discouraging 5 percent.[14]

In other nationally representative polls, in 1993 and again in 2005, Gallup pollsters asked respondents whether they would be more or less likely to donate their own or family members' organs after death if compensation were available. In both cases, 12 percent of respondents said they would be more likely to donate if financial incentives were offered, while 5 percent answered less likely—a margin of seven percentage points in favor of giving either their own or their deceased family members' organs.[15]

The 2005 version of the Gallup poll found similar results. Asked whether "payments would make them more likely" to donate their own organs, 17 percent answered in the affirmative, while 9 percent said they would be "less likely" to donate—a margin of eight percentage points in favor of giving. When asked about willingness to give a family member's organs, 19 percent answered "more likely," while 9 percent said "less likely," a margin of ten percentage points in favor of donation.

Notably, in both surveys, motivation to donate was highest among the youngest respondents. In 1993, 30 percent of eighteen- to twenty-four-year-olds surveyed said they would be "more likely" to donate their own organs for an incentive, while 7 percent said "less likely." For donation of family members' organs, the responses were 27 percent and 9 percent, respectively. In 2005, 34 percent of those eighteen to thirty-four years old said they would be more "more likely" to donate their own organs for payment, while only 6 percent said "less likely." The offer of incentives prompted 33 percent to say they would be "more likely" to give a family member's organs and 7 percent to say "less likely."[16]

Among polls of other populations, a 1999 survey of a random sample of 300 prospective jurors at the Philadelphia County Courthouse found that incentives markedly increased the intent to offer both deceased-donor and living-donor organs among respondents who had not planned to do so, more than they suppressed the intent to donate among those who had already believed they would do so.[17] The 2005 survey of Pennsylvania residents cited above found that attitudes of the majority were unchanged by the prospect of incentives, but among those who said that incentives made a difference, the net effect was to increase willingness to donate.[18]

For a 2006 report in *Transplantation*, researchers interviewed over 500 family members who had suffered the loss of a loved one within the previous few months and who, at that time, had been approached about donating the deceased's organs. Of individuals who had given consent, 61 percent said that they would not have done so had financial incentives been offered at the time. Conversely, 59 percent of those who refused to give consent when their loved died said that an offer of a financial incentive at the time would have led them to consent.[19] A study published in 2006 surveyed over 1,000 adults in Scotland and found that the proposal of a cash allowance of two thousand pounds toward crematorium costs or for charity enhanced willingness to donate at death by four or three times, respectively. The prospect of receiving a payment as a living donor encouraged more respondents than it discouraged, but by very little.[20]

In summary, the preponderance of survey evidence regarding the acceptability of incentives as motivators for donation, at both policy and personal levels, is positive. Younger cohorts seem to be especially receptive. None of the polls was designed to inquire about the acceptability of a donor compensation system in which all patients, not just the financially well-off who could afford to purchase organs, benefited. If those conditions had been presented to respondents, thereby allaying concerns about uneven distribution of organs, it is plausible that higher endorsement rates would have been obtained.[21]

Appendix D

Religious Considerations

Sally Satel

All of the major religions accept the practice of donating organs for transplantation, justifying it variously as a matter of conscience, an act of great love and charity, and a moral duty to save lives.[1] With the exception of some Orthodox Jews who do not accept the validity of brain death criteria, most religious leaders explicitly encourage voluntary donation from both living and newly deceased donors.[2]

Religious views about compensating organ donors are more diverse. Clerical leaders must grapple with ethical challenges posed by the potential exploitation of the poor, risks to buyers and sellers, and the possibility for mutilation of the donor's body in the absence of his or her medical gain.[3] This appendix describes the attitudes of Catholics, Muslims, and Jews toward compensated organ donation. These three major religious groups lie along a continuum of acceptance, with Jews being most open to the idea of donor compensation and Catholics the least.

Judaism

Many Jewish scholars accept the idea of rewarding people for donating organs for transplantation. Rabbi Shlomo Goren, the third Ashkenazi chief rabbi of Israel, writes that "the donation of a kidney in consideration of financial reward does not change its positive characteristic."[4] He continues, "We have no halachic basis [that is, no basis rooted in Jewish law] on which to prohibit one from donating a kidney in consideration of financial gain."

Abraham Sofer, expressing the view of Rabbi Shlomo Zalman Auerbach, writes, "One cannot say that a person who contributes his kidney in consideration of financial gain is doing something contemptible rather than praiseworthy. . . . [I]t remains most commendable even if his primary purpose was . . . to pay off his debt or obtain medical services for himself or his family members."[5] Yisrael Meir Lau, Ashkenazi chief rabbi from 1993 to 2003, affirms that Jewish law permits the sale of one's organs if their removal doesn't harm the seller's health; he likens the sale to receiving money to pay for one's medical expenses and suffering after being injured by another and concludes that "one who volunteers to be injured to save another does not forfeit similar compensation."[6] Rabbi Yosef Shalom Elyashiv, a leading halachic authority, says that selling organs is allowable as long as the seller's financial need is great enough to override the general prohibition in Jewish law against harming oneself.[7] In 2002, the *Israel Medical Association Journal* published a paper entitled "Legalizing the Sale of Kidneys for Transplantation: Suggested Guidelines," advocating a donor fee to be paid by the Israeli Ministry of Health.[8] Other scholars conclude that Jewish ethics allow organ sales, provided their purpose is to save life.[9]

Islam

Within the Islamic faith, the ethical status of organ donor compensation is complex. In the abstract, Muslim jurists generally condemn payment for organs because they believe God owns the human body and, therefore, humans do not have the right to sell organs they do not truly possess.[10] Most Shiite jurists and an increasing number of Sunni scholars believe, however, that life-threatening circumstances change the rules, and that organ trade is an acceptable means to save lives.[11] For example, a survey of thirty-two Muslim scholars found uniform agreement that organ trading is not permissible, yet 68.7 percent of them made an exception if the only alternative was death.[12]

This flexibility flows, in part, from the Islamic principle that necessity "makes what would otherwise be prohibited licit"[13]—the position endorsed by the Ad Hoc Administration of the Ministry of Waqfs and Islamic Affairs, which passed *fatwa* number 455/85 deeming purchase of an organ permissible if another's life is contingent upon it.[14] The *fatwa* (an Islamic and legal decree) reads as follows:

> As for the patient's purchase of a kidney from another person, the rule is that such act is impermissible, because Allah has honoured man, so it is not permitted to cut some of his organs and sell them at any price, whatsoever, but if the patient does not find a donor to give him his kidney, and his life is endangered, while he cannot find any other means to cure his illness, then purchase of organs is permissible, because the patient, then, is driven by a dire necessity.[15]

Mokhtar Al-Mahdi, chairman of the neurosurgery department at Ibn Sina Hospital in Kuwait, holds a similar view. "Until we can obtain an adequate supply of organs through voluntary and uncompensated donation," he writes, "we must countenance the possibility of offering to donors material recompense, on condition that no publicity in this respect is made."[16]

Muhammad Sayed Tantawi, the grand mufti of Egypt and a widely respected authority in Islamic jurisprudence, likewise declares that "man's sale of any of his organs is lawfully invalid and prohibited. Such sale is only permissible in the rarest cases decided by reliable doctors when they deem a patient's life contingent upon that sale."[17] Tantawi notes, however, that Muslim religious authorities hold differing views on the issue. He describes three classes of jurists: those who believe it is always unlawful to sell or donate organs; those who accept only donation, and only when it saves a life and does not harm the donor; and those who sanction compensation if paying for an organ is the only way to save a life.[18]

Yet another viewpoint is held by Muslim authorities in Iran, who have endorsed the broader permissibility of organ trade. Leading Shi'a clerics specify a variety of conditions under which organ transplantation is permissible. Those regulating transplant from a living person require that the patient's life is at stake; that, to the extent possible, the organ comes from a non-Muslim; and that the donor's life will not be jeopardized. As long as these conditions are met, "it is not unlikely that one be allowed to sell his organs in his lifetime."[19] Notably, Islamic Iran is the only country in the world in which organ sales are legal.[20] It is also the only Islamic country that permits vasectomy, tubal ligation, egg donation, embryo implantation, and first-trimester abortions in cases of emotional or physical harm to the mother or disease or malformation of the fetus.[21] As an Islamic country that observes and practices a flexible version of Shi'a Islam, Iran is unique in its embrace of medical technology.[22]

Catholicism

Perhaps the earliest consideration among Catholics of remuneration for a body part was expressed publicly by Pope Pius XII in 1956. In an address to the Italian Association of Donors of the Cornea, he asked,

> Is it necessary, as often happens, to refuse any compensation as a matter of principle? The question has arisen. Without doubt there can be grave abuses if recompense is demanded; but it would be an exaggeration to say that any acceptance or requirement of recompense is immoral. The case is analogous to that of blood transfusion; it is to the donor's credit if he refuses recompense, but it is not necessarily a fault to accept it.[23]

Half a century later, in 2000, Pope John Paul II declared that transplants were "a great step forward in science's service of man." He added:

> It must first be emphasized, as I observed on another occasion, that every organ transplant has its source in a decision of great ethical value: "the decision to offer without reward a part of one's own body for the health and well-being of another person". . . . Here precisely lies the nobility of the gesture, a gesture which is a genuine act of love.[24]

Having given organ transplants the highest moral accolades, the pope then warned against a potential for abuse: "Any procedure which tends to commercialize human organs or to consider them as items of exchange or trade must be considered morally unacceptable, because to use the body as an 'object' is to violate the dignity of the human person." A key aspect of ensuring dignity, he says, is "the need for informed consent . . the human 'authenticity' of such a decisive gesture requires that individuals be properly informed about the processes involved, in order to be in a position to consent or decline in a free and conscientious manner."[25]

The Catholic consensus position endorses Pope John Paul II's opposition to the commercialization of human organs. The United States Conference of Catholic Bishops issued a directive asserting that living donor transplantation is acceptable, but "economic advantages should not accrue to the donor."[26] The National Catholic Bioethics Center has stated the position even more forcefully, saying it "strongly opposes any regulated market of organ sales."[27]

Despite mainstream opposition to compensation for organ donation, some Catholic theologians and philosophers are trying to blaze a trail to an accommodation that would maintain the nobility of the donation while admitting of regulated forms of compensation consistent with the human dignity both of donor and recipient.[28] Philosopher Nicholas Capaldi, for instance, states in his article, "A Catholic Perspective on Organ Sales," that "there is no reason why any of the parties involved in the transactions need show disrespect for the divine origins of human life."[29]

Along similar lines, philosopher Mark J. Cherry argues that the Catholic principle of totality (the Thomist concept that a part of the body may be sacrificed to save the whole) is not violated by compensation because "the natural good of the individual's bodily functional wholeness is not set at risk."[30] Nor is Kant's moral imperative against treating other people solely as means to an end transgressed, Cherry says. Among other things, "Since persons are always to be treated as ends in themselves [referring to donors within a market], it is plausible that Kant could endorse the moral permissibility of organ selling as helping others to maintain personhood."[31] Furthermore, relinquishing a kidney in life can be justified if the compensation received is used to save the life of another, as in the case of a father who sells a kidney to pay for a vital operation for his child.[32]

Notes

Introduction

1. *Herald Sun* (Melbourne), "Dutch to Air Kidney Big Donor Reality Show," May 27, 2007, http://www.news.com.au/heraldsun/story/0,21985,21801522-663,00.html (accessed April 1, 2008).

2. *BBC News Online*, "TV Kidney Competition Was a Hoax," June 2, 2007, http://news.bbc.co.uk/2/hi/entertainment/6714063.stm (accessed March 20, 2008).

3. Organ Procurement and Transplantation Network, "Overall by Organ: Current U.S. Waiting List," http://www.optn.org/data (accessed April 2, 2008).

4. National Kidney Foundation, Kidney Disease Outcomes Quality Initiative, "Clinical Practice Guidelines for Chronic Kidney Disease," http://www.kidney.org/professionals/Kdoqi/guidelines_ckd/p6_comp_g12.htm (accessed February 6, 2008); Paul L. Kimmel and Samir S. Patel, "Quality of Life in Patients with Chronic Kidney Disease: Focus on End-Stage Renal Disease Treated with Hemodialysis," *Seminars in Nephrology* 26, no. 1 (January 2006): 68–79; for employment status data see U.S. Renal Data System (USRDS), "Percent Distribution of Patients, by Employment Status," *2007 ADR/Reference Tables*, table C.15.1 (supplement), http:www.usrds.org/reference.htm (accessed June 30, 2008); dialysis patient status broken out by Tara Rogan, research analyst USRDS, personal communication with the author, July 1, 2008 (data on file with the author).

5. Fernando G. Cosio, Amir Alamir, Susan Yim, Todd E. Pesavento, Michael E. Falkenhain, Mitchell L. Henry, Elmahdi A. Elkhammas, Elizabeth A. Davies, Ginny L. Bumgardner, and Ronald M. Ferguson, "Patient Survival after Renal Transplantation: I. The Impact of Dialysis Pre-Transplant," *Kidney International* 53, no. 3 (March 1998): 767–72; Herwig-Ulf Meier-Kriesche, Friedrich K. Port, Akinlolu O. Ojo, Steven M. Rudich, Julie A. Hanson, Diane M. Cibrik, Alan B. Leichtman, and Bruce Kaplan, "Effect of Waiting Time on Renal Transplant Outcome," *Kidney International* 58, no. 3 (September 2000): 1311–17; Seema Baid-Agrawal and Ulrich Frei, "Living Donor Renal Transplantation: Recent Developments and Perspectives," *Nature Clinical Practice Nephrology* 3, no. 1 (January 2007): 31, 39; Kevin C. Mange, Marshall M. Joffe, and Harold I. Feldman, "Effect of the Use or Nonuse of Long-Term Dialysis on the Subsequent Survival of Renal Transplants from Living Donors," *New England Journal of*

Medicine 344, no. 10 (March 2001): 726–31. The median five-year survival rate for a new dialysis-dependent patient is 35 percent, compared to 75 percent after kidney transplantation. U.S. Renal Data System, "Adjusted Five-Year Survival, by Modality & Primary Diagnosis," *2008 Annual Data Report*, figure 6.10, http://www.usrds.org/2008/pdf/v2_06_2008.pdf (accessed October 23, 2008).

6. Benjamin Hippen, "Preventive Measures May Not Reduce the Demand for Kidney Transplantation. There Is Reason to Suppose This Is Not the Case," *Kidney International* 70, no. 3 (August 2006): 606–7; A. O. Ojo, J. A. Hanson, H. Meier-Kriesche, C. N. Okechukwu, R. A. Wolfe, A. B. Leichtman, et al., "Survival in Recipients of Marginal Cadaveric Donor Kidneys Compared with Other Recipients and Wait-Listed Transplant Candidates," *Journal of the American Society of Nephrology* 12, no. 3 (March 2001): 589–97; R. M. Merion, V. B. Ashby, R. A. Wolfe, D. A. Distant, T. E. Hulbert-Shearon, R. A. Metzger, et al., "Deceased-Donor Characteristics and the Survival Benefit of Kidney Transplantation," *Journal of the American Medical Association* 294, no. 21 (December 7, 2005): 2726–33.

7. Organ Procurement and Transplantation Network, "Death Removals by Year by Diagnosis," national data, for kidneys, http://www.optn.org/latestData/rptData.asp (accessed June 26, 2008).

8. R. A. Stein, "Third of Patients on Transplant List Are Not Eligible," *Washington Post*, March 22, 2008, A01.

9. Jay L. Xue, Jennie Z. Ma, Thomas A. Louis, and Allan J. Collins, "Forecast of the Number of Patients with End-Stage Renal Disease in the United States to the Year 2010," *Journal of the American Society of Nephrology* 12, no. 12 (2001): 2753–58; Ojo et al., "Survival in Recipients"; Merion et al., "Deceased-Donor Characteristics."

10. U.S. Department of Health and Human Services, Centers for Disease Control and Prevention, "Hospitalization Discharge Diagnoses for Kidney Disease: United States, 1980–2005," *Morbidity and Mortality Weekly Report* 57, no. 12 (March 28, 2008): 309–12, http://www.cdc.gov/mmwR/PDF/wk/mm5712.pdf (accessed April 1, 2008). Counterintuitive as it may seem, preventive medicine may actually make things worse. As it stands now, the vast majority of people with kidney disease die from complications of heart disease and stroke before ever progressing to renal failure. But as the treatment of heart attacks, strokes, hypertension, and diabetes is improving, the natural history of these diseases is evolving as well, and those afflicted are living longer—long enough to develop renal failure. See Hippen, "Preventive Measures May Not Reduce Demand."

11. Jesse D. Schold, Titte R. Srinivas, Liise K. Kayler, and Herwig-Ulf Meier-Kriesche, "The Overlapping Risk Profile between Dialysis Patients Listed and Not Listed for Renal Transplantation," *American Journal of Transplantation* 8, no. 1 (January 2008): 58–68.

12. G. E. W. Wolstenholme and Maeve O'Conner, eds., *Ethics in Medical Progress: With Special Reference to Transplantation* (London: J & A Churchill, 1966), 35; Jesse Dukeminier Jr., "Supplying Organs for Transplantation," *Michigan Law Review* 68, no. 5 (April 1970): 811–66; Simon Rottenberg, "The Production and Exchange of Body Parts," in *Towards Liberty: Essays in Honor of Ludwig von Mises on the Occasion of his 90th Birthday*,

September 29, 1971, ed. Friedrich A. von Hayek (Menlo Park, Calif.: Institute for Humane Studies, 1971), 326; Timothy M. Hartman, "The Buying and Selling of Human Organs From the Living: Why Not?" *Akron Law Review* 13, no. 1 (1979): 152–74; Marvin Brams, "Transplantable Human Organs: Should Their Sale Be Authorized by State Statutes?" *American Journal of Law and Medicine* 2, no. 3 (Summer 1977): 183–95; Harry Schwartz, "Providing Incentives for Organ Donations," *Wall Street Journal*, July 25, 1983, 10.

13. Margaret Engel, "Va. Doctor Plans Company to Arrange Sale of Human Kidneys," *Washington Post,* September 19, 1983, A9. See chapter 8 and appendix A.

14. Susan H. Denise, "Regulating the Sale of Human Organs," *Virginia Law Review* 71, no. 6 (September 1985): 1015–38.

15. National Organ Transplant Act (NOTA), Pub. L. No. 98–507, sec. 301 (1984) § 274e. For an explanation of the statute's wording regarding interstate commerce, see chapter 8, note 13. With the enactment in 2007 of H.R. 710 (the Charlie W. Norwood Living Organ Donation Act), section (a) was amended to read: The preceding sentence does not apply with respect to human organ paired donation

16. Office of Legal Counsel, U.S. Department of Justice, "Legality of Alternative Organ Donation Practices under 42 U.S.C. § 274e," March 28, 2007, http://www.usdoj.gov/olc/2007/organtransplant.pdf; U.S. House of Representatives, Committee on Energy and Commerce, Subcommittee on Health and the Environment, *Hearings on the National Organ Transplant Act*, 98th Cong., 1st sess., July 1983, statement of Representative Albert Gore Jr., 9–10. The text reads, "The National Center for Human Organ Acquisition would report annually on the status of voluntary organ donation. If the center judges efforts to improve voluntary donation are unsuccessful, consideration in progressing fashion would be given to the following: First, provision of incentives, such as a voucher system or tax credit for a donor's estate; Second, a system of mandated choice such as requiring selection of donor status, yes or no, at time of driver's license issuance. In other words, it would remain completely and totally voluntary, but the choice would have to be made yes or no. Third, adoption of a system of presumed consent unless objection is registered in advance."

17. Ellen Sheehy, Suzanne L. Conrad, Lori E. Brigham, Richard Luskin, Phyllis Weber, Mark Eakin, Lawrence Schkade, and Lawrence Hunsicker, "Estimating the Number of Potential Organ Donors in the United States," *New England Journal of Medicine* 349, no. 7 (August 2003): 667–74.

18. Committee on Increasing Rates of Organ Donation, *Organ Donation: Opportunities for Action*, ed. James F. Childress, and Catharyn T. Liverman, (Washington, D.C.: National Academies Press, 2006), 100, table 4-1; see Organ Procurement and Transplantation Network, "Donors Recovered in the U.S. by Donor Type," http://www.optn.org/data (accessed March 1, 2008).

19. Presumed Consent Foundation Inc., "Solutions," http://www.presumed consent.org/solutions.htm (accessed March 4, 2008). Furthermore, while European countries with presumed-consent (also known as opt-out) policies did enjoy a boost in cadaver kidneys after the policy was implemented, it is unclear whether their success was

due to the new policy itself or to the simultaneous investment made in procurement infrastructure. To be sure, a presumed-consent strategy has merit. Another plan known as "forward" payment (wherein individuals arrange to have their organs taken at death in exchange for a payment to their estates or families) is also worth considering, but is beyond the scope of this book. See Kieran Healy, "Do Presumed Consent Laws Raise Organ Procurement Rates?" *De Paul Law Review* 55, no. 3 (Spring 2006): 1017–44.

20. Mark Reiner, Danielle Cornell, and Richard J. Howard, "Development of a Successful Non-Heart-Beating Organ Donation Program," *Progress in Transplantation* 13, no. 3 (September 2003): 225–31.

21. Katarina Anderson, data analyst, United Network for Organ Sharing, personal communication with the author, February 11, 2008. In 2006, the Organ Procurement Transplant Network projected that the number of donors after cardiac death could be only 2,018 by the year 2013; a salutary contribution, of course, but quite modest compared to predicted demand. See Organ Procurement and Transplantation Network and United Network for Organ Sharing, "Progress towards the HRSA Donor-Related Program Goals," September 2006, http://www.optn.org/SharedContentDocuments/Board_handout_sept2006_REVISED_OCT.pdf (accessed April 1, 2008).

22. Connie L. Davis and Francis L. Delmonico, "Living-Donor Kidney Transplantation: A Review of Current Practices for the Live Donor," *Journal of the American Society of Nephrology* 16, no. 7 (July 2005): 2098–2110. Fifteen to twenty years after transplantation, half of all kidneys obtained from a living donor are still functioning well, compared to ten to twelve years for a kidney from a deceased donor. See Robert Gaston, "Improving Access to Renal Transplantation," *Seminars in Dialysis* 18, no. 6 (November 2005): 482–86; Ojo et al., "Survival in Recipients"; Friedrich K. Port, Jennifer L. Bragg, Robert A. Metzger, Dawn M. Dykstra, Brenda W. Gillespie, Eric W. Young, Francis L. Delmonico, James J. Wynn, Robert M. Merion, Robert A. Wolfe, and Philip J. Held, "Donor Characteristics Associated with Reduced Graft Survival: An Approach to Expanding the Pool of Kidney Donors," *Transplantation* 74, no. 9 (November 2002): 1281–86; Mark A. Schnitzler, James F. Whiting, Daniel C. Brennan, Grace Lin, Will Chapman, Jeffrey Lowell, Stuart Boxerman, Karen L. Hardinger, and Zoltan Kalo, "The Expanded Criteria Donor Dilemma in Cadaveric Renal Transplantation," *Transplantation* 75, no. 12 (June 2003): 1940–45; James F. Whiting, Robert S. Woodward, Edward Y. Zavala, David S. Cohen, Jill E. Martin, Gary G. Singer, Jeffrey A. Lowell, M. Roy First, Daniel C. Brennan, and Mark A. Schnitzler, "Economic Costs of Expanded Criteria Donors in Cadaveric Renal Transplantation: Analysis of Medicare Payments," *Transplantation* 70, no. 5 (September 2000): 755–60.

23. In 2005, 6.4 percent of the Medicare budget was spent on behalf of 0.6 percent of eligible Medicare beneficiaries; see U.S. Renal Data System, "2007 Annual Data Report: Costs of ESAs in CKD & ESRD Patients," figure 11.1, http://www.usrds.org/2007/view/11_econ.asp (accessed October 3, 2007). Of that $21 billion, only $0.586 billion was spent on kidney acquisition and transplantation costs. U.S. Renal Data System, "Total Medicare Expenditures, by Modality," *2007 Annual Data Report*, figure 11.7, http://www.usrds.org/2007/view/11_econ.asp (accessed October 3, 2007).

24. In some instances, a loved one wants to donate but is not biologically compatible with the patient. If this couple can trade with another mismatched couple, the transplants can take place: The donor from couple A gives a kidney to the compatible recipient of couple B, and vice versa. The virtue is that two lives are saved instead of none. Without the paired exchange, both patients would languish on dialysis. Perhaps six thousand such pairs exist now, and one thousand new ones are expected annually. Another, more unusual, arrangement is called a donor chain, in which an anonymous living donor gives a kidney to someone on the UNOS waiting list. That person's incompatible donor gives his or her organ to one-half of another incompatible pair, and so on, in domino fashion. These exchanges are a welcome innovation, but they provide, at most, a partial solution. Dorry L. Segev, Sommer E. Gentry, Daniel S. Warren, Brigitte Reeb, and Robert A. Montgomery, "Kidney Paired Donation and Optimizing the Use of Live Donor Organs," *Journal of the American Medical Association* 293, no. 15 (April 2005): 1883–90; Sommer E. Gentry, Dorry L. Segev, and Robert A. Montgomery, "A Comparison of Populations Served by Kidney Paired Donation and List Paired Donation," *American Journal of Transplantation* 5, no. 8 (August 2005): 1914–21; Weill Cornell Medical College, "Kidney Transplant Chain Initiated at New York–Presbyterian/Weill Cornell," press release, February 20, 2008, http://news.med.cornell.edu/wcmc/wcmc_2008/02_20_08.shtml (accessed April 1, 2008).

25. Barbara Feder Ostrov, "Transplant Dilemma Grows," *San Jose Mercury News*, November 26, 2006.

Chapter 1: Risks of Kidney Transplantation to a Living Donor

1. R. W. Evans, D. L. Manninen, et al., "The Quality of Life of Patients with End-Stage Renal Disease," *New England Journal of Medicine* 312, no. 9 (1985): 553–59; R. A. Wolfe, V. B. Ashby, et al., "Comparison of Mortality in All Patients on Dialysis, Patients on Dialysis Awaiting Transplantation, and Recipients of a First Cadaveric Transplant," *New England Journal of Medicine* 341, no. 23 (1999): 1725–30; P. Schnuelle, D. Lorenz, et al., "Impact of Renal Cadaveric Transplantation on Survival in End-Stage Renal Failure: Evidence for Reduced Mortality Risk Compared with Hemodialysis during Long-Term Follow-Up," *Journal of the American Society of Nephrology* 9, no. 11 (1998): 2135–41.

2. Fernando G. Cosio, Amir Alamir, Susan Yim, Todd E. Pesavento, Michael E. Falkenhain, Mitchell L. Henry, Elmahdi A. Elkhammas, Elizabeth A. Davies, Ginny L. Bumgardner, and Ronald M. Ferguson, "Patient Survival after Renal Transplantation. I. The Impact of Dialysis Pre-Transplant," *Kidney International* 53, no. 3 (1998): 767–72; H. U. Meier-Kreische, F. K. Port, et al., "Effect of Waiting Time on Renal Transplant Outcome," *Kidney International* 58, no. 3 (2000): 1311–17.

3. Jay L. Xue, Jennie Z. Ma, Thomas A. Louis, and Allan J. Collins, "Forecast of the Number of Patients with End-Stage Renal Disease in the United States to the Year 2010," *Journal of the American Society of Nephrology* 12, no. 12 (2001): 2753–58.

4. Ibid.

5. A. O. Ojo, J. A. Hanson, H. Meier-Kriesche, C. N. Okechukwu, R. A. Wolfe, A. B. Leichtman, et al., "Survival in Recipients of Marginal Cadaveric Donor Kidneys Compared with Other Recipients and Wait-Listed Transplant Patients," *Journal of the American Society of Nephrology* 12, no. 3 (2001): 589–97.

6. R. M. Merion, V. B. Ashby, R. A. Wolfe, D. A. Distant, T. E. Hulbert-Shearon, R. A. Metzger, et al., "Deceased-Donor Characteristics and the Survival Benefit of Kidney Transplantation," *JAMA* 294, no. 21 (2005): 2726–33.

7. Antigens are naturally occurring proteins on the surface of the tissues.

8. A website called livingdonorsonline.org, initiated by a kidney donor who saw a need for better dissemination of information, is an extremely informative resource for prospective donors.

9. William H. Bay and Lee A. Hebert, "The Living Donor in Kidney Transplantation," *Annals of Internal Medicine* 106, no. 5 (1987): 719–27; J. S. Najarian, B. M. Chavers, et al., "20 Years or More of Follow-Up of Living Kidney Donors," *Lancet* 340, no. 8823 (1992): 807–10; Arthur J. Matas, Stephen T. Bartlett, Alan B. Leichtman, and Francis L. Delmonico, "Morbidity and Mortality after Living Kidney Donation in 1999–2001: A Survey of United States Transplant Centers," *American Journal of Transplantation* 3, no. 7 (2003): 830–34.

10. A. L. Friedman, T. G. Peters, K. W. Jones, et al. "Fatal and Nonfatal Hemorrhagic Complications of Living Kidney Donation," *Annals of Surgery* 243 (2006): 126–30.

11. Bay and Hebert noted an overall major complication rate of 1.8 percent after open nephrectomy. Bay and Hebert, "The Living Donor in Kidney Transplantation." More recently, Johnson and others studied 871 open nephrectomy donors at the University of Minnesota and reported that 8.6 percent had complications, only 0.2 percent of which, however (two cases), were considered major. E. M. Johnson, M. J. Remucal, et al., "Complications and Risks of Living Donor Nephrectomy," *Transplantation* 64, no. 8 (1997): 1124–28.

12. L. M. Su, L. E. Ratner, and R. A. Montgomery, "Laparoscopic Live Donor Nephrectomy: Trends in Donor and Recipient Morbidity Following 381 Consecutive Cases," *Annals of Surgery* 240 (2004): 427–32.

13. Sixteen days for laparoscopic versus fifty-one days for open nephrectomy.

14. Stephen T. Bartlett and Eugene J. Schweitzer, "Laparoscopic Living Donor Nephrectomy for Kidney Transplantation," *Dialysis & Transplantation* 28, no. 6 (1999): 318–31.

15. The aorta and the inferior vena cava.

16. I. Fehrman-Ekholm, C. G. Elinder, et al., "Kidney Donors Live Longer," *Transplantation* 64, no. 7 (1997): 976–78.

17. B. Andersen, J. B. Hansen, and S. J. Jorgensen, "Survival after Nephrectomy," *Scandinavian Journal of Urology and Nephrology* 2, no. 2 (1968): 91–94.

18. Ibid.; N. B. Shulman, C. E. Ford, et al., "Prognostic Value of Serum Creatinine and Effect of Treatment of Hypertension on Renal Function. Results from the Hypertension

Detection and Follow-Up Program," *Hypertension* 13, no. 5 supp. (1989): I-80–93; E. M. Damsgaard, A. Froland, et al., "Microalbuminuria as Predictor of Increased Mortality in Elderly People," *British Medical Journal* 300, no. 6720 (1990): 297–300; P. J. Friedman, "Serum Creatinine: An Independent Predictor of Survival after Stroke," *Journal of Internal Medicine* 229, no. 2 (1991): 175–79; A. D. Hamdan, F. B. Pomposelli Jr., et al., "Renal Insufficiency and Altered Postoperative Risk in Carotid Endarterectomy," *Journal of Vascular Surgery* 29, no. 6 (1999): 1006–11; J. P. Matts, J. N. Karnegis, et al., "Serum Creatinine as an Independent Predictor of Coronary Heart Disease Mortality in Normotensive Survivors of Myocardial Infarction," *Journal of Family Practice* 36, no. 5 (1993): 497–503; D. L. Dries, D. V. Exner, et al., "The Prognostic Implications of Renal Insufficiency in Asymptomatic and Symptomatic Patients with Left Ventricular Dysfunction," *Journal of the American College of Cardiology* 35, no. 3 (2000): 681–89; R. J. Anderson, M. O'Brien, et al., "Mild Renal Failure Is Associated with Adverse Outcome after Cardiac Valve Surgery," *American Journal of Kidney Diseases* 35, no. 6 (2000): 1127–34; D. E. Weiner, H. Tighiouart, et al., "Kidney Disease as a Risk Factor for Recurrent Cardiovascular Disease and Mortality," *American Journal of Kidney Diseases* 44, no. 2 (2004): 198–206; L. F. Fried, M. G. Shlipak, et al., "Renal Insufficiency as a Predictor of Cardiovascular Outcomes and Mortality in Elderly Individuals," *Journal of the American College of Cardiology* 41 (2003): 1364–72; R. M. Henry, P. J. Kostense, et al., "Mild Renal Insufficiency Is Associated with Increased Cardiovascular Mortality: The Hoorn Study," *Kidney International* 62 (2002): 1402–7; P. Muntner, J. He, et al., "Renal Insufficiency and Subsequent Death Resulting from Cardiovascular Disease in the United States," *Journal of the American Society of Nephrology* 13 (2002): 745–53; S. G. Wannamethee, A. G. Shaper, and I. J. Perry, "Serum Creatinine Concentration and Risk of Cardiovascular Disease: A Possible Marker for Increased Risk of Stroke," *Stroke* 28, no. 3 (1997): 557–63; B. F. Culleton, M. G. Larson, et al., "Cardiovascular Disease and Mortality in a Community-Based Cohort with Mild Renal Insufficiency," *Kidney International* 56, no. 6 (1999): 2214–19; G. Manjunath, H. Tighiouart, et al., "Level of Kidney Function as a Risk Factor for Atherosclerotic Cardiovascular Outcomes in the Community," *Journal of the American College of Cardiology* 41, no. 1 (2003): 47–55; A. S. Go, G. M. Cherton, et al., "Chronic Kidney Disease and the Risks of Death, Cardiovascular Events, and Hospitalization," *New England Journal of Medicine* 351, no. 13 (2004): 1296–1305; R. N. Foley, A. M. Murray, et al., "Chronic Kidney Disease and the Risk for Cardiovascular Disease, Renal Replacement and Death in the United States Medicare Population, 1998 to 1999," *Journal of the American Society of Nephrology* 16, no. 2 (2005): 489–95; A. X. Garg, W. F. Clark, et al., "Moderate Renal Insufficiency and the Risk of Cardiovascular Mortality: Results from the NHANES I," *Kidney International* 61, no. 4 (2002): 1486–94.

19. Najarian, Chavers, et al., "20 Years or More of Follow-Up of Living Kidney Donors"; R. C. Pabico, B. A. McKenna, and R. B. Freeman, "Renal Function Before and After Unilateral Nephrectomy in Renal Donors," *Kidney International* 8, no. 3 (1975): 166–75; P. M. ter Wee, A. M. Tegess, and A. J. Donker, "Renal Reserve Filtration Capacity Before

and After Kidney Donation," *Journal of Internal Medicine* 228, no. 4 (1990): 393–99; R. G. Anderson, A. J. Bueschen, L. K. Lloyd, et al., "Short-Term and Long-Term Changes in Renal Function after Donor Nephrectomy," *Journal of Urology* 145, no. 1 (1991): 11–13; I. Penn, C. G. Halgrimson, et al., "Use of Living Donors in Kidney Transplantation in Man," *Archives of Surgery* 101, no. 2 (1970): 226–31; J. M. Davison, P. R. Uldall, and J. Walls, "Renal Function Studies after Nephrectomy in Renal Donors" *British Medical Journal* 1, no. 6017 (1976): 1050–52; O. Ringden, L. Friman, et al., "Living Related Kidney Donors: Complications and Long-Term Renal Function," *Transplantation* 25, no. 4 (1978): 221–23; S. Dean, C. J. Rudge, and M. Joyce, "Live Related Renal Transplantation: An Analysis of 141 Donors," *Transplant Proceedings* 14 (1982): 657; F. Vincenti, W. J. Amend Jr., et al., "Long-Term Renal Function in Kidney Donors. Sustained Compensatory Hyperfiltration with No Adverse Effects," *Transplantation* 36, no. 6 (1983): 626–29; D. Weiland, D. E. R. Sutherland, et al., "Information on 628 Living-Related Kidney Donors at a Single Institution, with Long-Term Follow-Up in 472 Cases," *Transplant Proceedings* 16 (1984): 5; R. M. Hakim, R. C. Goldszer, and B. M. Brenner, "Hypertension and Proteinuria: Long-Term Sequelae of Uninephrectomy in Humans," *Kidney International* 25, no. 6 (1984): 930–36; I. J. Miller, M. Suthanthiran, et al., "Impact of Renal Donation. Long-Term Clinical and Biochemical Follow-Up of Living Donors in a Single Center," *American Journal of Medicine* 79, no. 2 (1985): 201–8; J. S. Tapson, S. M. Marshall, et al., "Renal Function and Blood Pressure after Donor Nephrectomy," *Proceedings of the European Dialysis and Transplant Association–European Renal Association* 21 (1985): 580–7; C. F. Anderson, J. A. Velosa, et al. "The Risks of Unilateral Nephrectomy: Status of Kidney Donors 10 to 20 Years Postoperatively," *Mayo Clinic Proceedings* 60, no. 6 (1985): 367–74; L. L. Bohannon, J. M. Barry, et al., "Renal Function 27 Years after Unilateral Nephrectomy for Related Donor Kidney Transplantation," *Journal of Urology* 140, no. 4 (1988): 810–11; A. J. Hoitsma, L. C. Paul, et al., "Long Term Follow-Up of Living Kidney Donors. A Two-Centre Study," *Netherlands Journal of Medicine* 28, no. 6 (1985): 226–30; M. Sobh, A. Nabeeh, et al., "Long-Term Follow-Up of the Remaining Kidney in Living Related Kidney Donors," *International Urology and Nephrology* 21, no. 5 (1989): 547–53; O. Mathillas, P. O. Attman, et al., "Proteinuria and Renal Function in Kidney Transplant Donors 10–18 Years after Donor Uninephrectomy," *Upsala Journal of Medical Sciences* 90, no. 1 (1985): 37–42; J. S. Tapson, "End-Stage Renal Failure after Donor Nephrectomy," *Nephron* 42, no. 3 (1986): 262–64; J. Ladefoged, "Renal Failure 22 Years after Kidney Donation," *Lancet* 339, no. 8785 (1992): 124–25; S. Smith, P. Laprad, and J. Grantham, "Long-Term Effect of Uninephrectomy on Serum Creatinine Concentration and Arterial Blood Pressure," *American Journal of Kidney Diseases* 6, no. 3 (1985): 143–48; D. O'Donnell, J. Seggie, et al., "Renal Function after Nephrectomy for Donor Organs," *South African Medical Journal* 69, no. 3 (1986): 177–79; T. Talseth, P. Fauchald, et al., "Long-Term Blood Pressure and Renal Function in Kidney Donors," *Kidney International* 29, no. 5 (1986): 1072–76; S. L. Williams, J. Oler, and D. K. Jorkasky, "Long-Term Renal Function in Kidney Donors: A Comparison of Donors and Their Siblings," *Annals of Internal Medicine* 105, no. 1 (1986):

1–8; D. A. Goldfarb, S. F. Matin, et al., "Renal Outcome 25 Years after Donor Nephrectomy," *Journal of Urology* 166, no. 6 (2001): 2043–47; J. F. Dunn, W. A. Nylander Jr., et al., "Living Related Kidney Donors: A 14-Year Experience," *Annals of Surgery* 203, no. 6 (1986): 637–43; T. Ramcharan and A. J. Matas, "Long-Term (20–37 Years) Follow-Up of Living Kidney Donors," *American Journal of Transplantation* 2, no. 10 (2002): 959–64; V. E. Torres, K. P. Offord, et al., "Blood Pressure Determinants in Living-Related Renal Allograft Donors and Their Recipients," *Kidney International* 31, no. 6 (1987): 1383–90; I. Fehrman-Ekholm, G. Nordén, et al., "Incidence of End-Stage Renal Disease among Live Kidney Donors," *Transplantation* 82, no. 12 (2006): 1646–48, reviewed in B. L. Kasiske, J. Z. Ma, et al., "Long-Term Effects of Reduced Renal Mass in Humans," *Kidney International* 48, no. 3 (1995): 814–19.

20. J. V. Donadio Jr., C. D. Farmer, et al., "Renal Function in Donors and Recipients of Renal Allotransplantation: Radioisotopic Measurements," *Annals of Internal Medicine* 66, no. 1 (1967): 105–15; A. G. Krohn, D. A. Ogden, and J. H. Holmes, "Renal Function in 29 Healthy Adults Before and After Nephrectomy," *JAMA* 196, no. 4 (1966): 322–24; W. J. Flanigan, R. O. Burns, et al., "Serial Studies of Glomerular Filtration Rate and Renal Plasma Flow in Kidney Transplant Donors, Identical Twins, and Allograft Recipients," *American Journal of Surgery* 116, no. 5 (1968): 788–94; G. Boner, W. D. Shelp, et al., "Factors Influencing the Increase in Glomerular Filtration Rate in the Remaining Kidney of Transplant Donors," *American Journal of Medicine* 55, no. 2 (1973): 169–74; Pabico, McKenna, and Freeman, "Renal Function Before and After Unilateral Nephrectomy"; Ter Wee, Tegzess, and Donker, "Renal Reserve Filtration Capacity Before and After Kidney Donation"; Anderson, Bueschen, Lloyd, et al., "Short-Term and Long-Term Changes in Renal Function"; A. Chanutin and E. G. Ferris, "Experimental Renal Insufficiency Produced by Partial Nephrectomy," *Archives of Internal Medicine* 49 (1932): 767.

21. Dunn, Nylander Jr., et al., "Living Related Kidney Donors"; Ramcharan and Matas, "Long-Term (20–37 Years) Follow-Up of Living Kidney Donors."

22. A. Spital, "Life Insurance for Kidney Donors—An Update," *Transplantation* 45, no. 4 (1988): 819–20.

23. Ellison et al. reported fifty-six living donors who had subsequently listed themselves on the national United Network for Organ Sharing waiting list in search of deceased-donor kidneys. Some had given their kidneys before the establishment of the UNOS database, making it difficult to determine the total number of living donors and thereby calculate the incidence of kidney failure among them. Even if such a calculation were possible, it might still underestimate the incidence of end-stage disease in living donors because those undergoing living-donor transplants and those developing renal failure but not listed for transplants would be overlooked in the calculation. In the Ellison report, 86 percent of the living donors who were later listed for transplants themselves had donated. M. D. Ellison, M. A. McBride, et al., "Living Kidney Donors in Need of Kidney Transplants: A Report from the Organ Procurement and Transplantation Network," *Transplantation* 74, no. 9 (2002): 1349–51.

24. Range, twenty-one to twenty-nine years; Najarian, Chavers, et al., "20 Years or More of Follow-Up of Living Kidney Donors."

25. Among those who returned questionnaires, mean age at time of donation was 43±1 years; range, sixteen to seventy years.

26. The measures were mean serum creatinine level, mean blood urea nitrogen, and mean creatinine clearance.

27. The characteristics were renal function, percentage taking antihypertensive medications, and percentage with proteinuria.

28. T. Ramcharan and A. J. Matas, "Long-Term (20–37 Years) Follow-Up of Living Kidney Donors," *American Journal of Transplantation* 2, no. 10 (2002): 959–64.

29. Of these 380, 124 reported no kidney problems and underwent no other testing. Of the remaining 256, 125 included records of their medical histories and physical examinations done by their local physicians, or laboratory test results; some included both medical records and test results.

30. Of the twenty-seven out of eighty-four for whom the cause of death was available, twenty-four had no renal disease, but three were on dialysis at the time of death. Of the three who died on dialysis, one had developed diabetes (which damaged the kidneys) and subsequent renal failure; another had developed renal failure secondary to a rare bleeding disorder at age seventy-six (thirty-two years after donation); and the third had developed renal failure as a result of cardiac disease.

31. Mean ± SD, 25 ± 3 years. Goldfarb, Matin, et al., "Renal Outcome 25 Years after Donor Nephrectomy."

32. Fehrman-Ekholm, G. Nordén, et al., "Incidence of End-Stage Renal Disease among Live Kidney Donors." The median follow-up was fourteen years; range, one to forty years.

33. Population studies have shown that elevated blood glucose levels (which are present in diabetics) and high blood pressure are both associated with an increased risk of proteinuria. M. Tozawa, K. Iseki, et al., "Influence of Smoking and Obesity on the Development of Proteinuria," *Kidney International* 62 (2002): 956–62; T. J. Watnick, R. R. Jenkins, et al., "Microalbuminuria and Hypertension in Long-Term Renal Donors," *Transplantation* 45, no. 1 (1988): 59–65; E. M. Briganti, P. Branley, et al., "Smoking Is Associated with Renal Impairment and Proteinuria in the Normal Population: The Ausdiab Kidney Study: Australian Diabetes, Obesity and Lifestyle Study," *American Journal of Kidney Diseases* 40 (2002): 704–12; K. Iseki, C. Iseki, et al., "Risk of Developing End-Stage Renal Disease in a Cohort of Mass Screening," *Kidney International* 49: 800–805; K. Iseki, Y. Ikemiya, et al., "Proteinuria and the Risk of Developing End-Stage Renal Disease," *Kidney International* 63 (2003):1468–74; K. Lhotta, H. J. Rumpelt, et al., "Cigarette Smoking and Vascular Pathology in Renal Biopsies," *Kidney International* 61 (2002): 648–54; M. Praga, E. Hernandez, et al., "Influence of Obesity on the Appearance of Proteinuria and Renal Insufficiency after Unilateral Nephrectomy," *Kidney International* 58 (2000): 2111–18, reviewed in R. Fattor, F. Silva, et al., "Effect of Unilateral Nephrectomy on Three Patients with Histopathological Evidence of Diabetic

Glomerulosclerosis in the Resected Kidney," *Journal of Diabetic Complications* 1, no. 3 (1987): 107–13.

34. M. Praga, E. Hernandez, et al., "Influence of Obesity on the Appearance of Proteinuria."

35. Body mass index ≥ 30.

36. Keep in mind, however, that this study overstates the probability of proteinuria for kidney donors, since its nondonor subjects likely had a serious disease requiring the nephrectomy and were not extensively screened to make sure their other kidney was normal. Living donors, in contrast, may be more thoroughly evaluated before being approved for the surgery.

37. Ramcharan and Matas, "Long-Term (20–37 Years) Follow-Up of Living Kidney Donors."

38. Muntner, He, et al., "Renal Insufficiency and Subsequent Death Resulting from Cardiovascular Disease in the United States"; J. M. Kaufman, N. J. Siegel, and J. P. Hayslett, "Functional and Hemodynamic Adaptation to Progressive Renal Ablation," *Circulation Research* 36, no. 2 (1975): 286–93; Fattor, Silva, et al., "Effect of Unilateral Nephrectomy on Three Patients"; M. J. Sampson and P. L. Drury, "Development of Nephropathy in Diabetic Patients with a Single Kidney," *Diabetic Medicine* 7 (1990): 258–60; S. P. Silveiro, L. A. DaCosta, et al., "Urinary Albumin Excretion Rate and Glomerular Filtration Rate in Single-Kidney Type Two Diabetic Patients," *Diabetes Care* 21, no. 9 (1998): 1521–24; M. Zeier, S. Geberth, et al., "The Effect of Uninephrectomy on Progression of Renal Failure in Autosomal Dominant Polycystic Kidney Disease," *Journal of the American Society of Nephrology* 3, no. 5 (1992): 1119–23.

39. E. Johnson, K. Anderson, et al., "Long-Term Follow-Up of Living Kidney Donors: Quality of Life After Donation," *Transplantation* 67: 717–21; G. C. Smith, T. Trauer, P. Kerr, and S. Chadban, "Prospective Psychosocial Monitoring of Living Kidney Donors Using the Short Form-36 Health Survey: Results at 12 Months," *Transplantation* 78 (2004): 1384–88; M. Jordan-Marsh, "The SF-36 Quality of Life Instrument: Updates and Strategies for Critical Care Research," *Critical Care Nurse* 22 (2002): 35–43; W. De Graaf Olson and A. Bogetti-Dumlao, "Living Donors' Perception of Their Quality of Health after Donation," *Progress in Transplantation* 11 (2001): 108–15; L. Schover, S. Streem, et al., "The Psychosocial Impact of Donating a Kidney: Long-Term Followup from a Urology Based Center," *Journal of Urology* 157 (1997):1596–1601; J. Buell, L. Lee, et al., "Laparoscopic Donor Nephrectomy vs. Open Live Donor Nephrectomy: A Quality of Life and Functional Study," *Clinical Transplantation* 19 (2005): 102–9; S. Isotani, M. Fujisawa, et al., "Quality of Life of Living Kidney Donors: The Short Form 36-Item Health Questionnaire Survey," *Urology* 60 (2002): 588; L. Westlie, P. Fawchald, et al., "Quality of Life in Norwegian Kidney Donors," *Nephrology Dialysis Transplantation* 8 (1993): 1146–50; M. Giessing, S. Reuter, et al., "Quality of Life of Living Kidney Donors in Germany: A Survey with the Validated Short Form-36 and Giessen Subjective Complaints List-24 Questionnaires," *Transplantation* 27 (2004): 786–87; C. Chen, Y. Chen, et al., "Risks and Quality of Life Changes in Living Kidney Donors,"

Transplantation Proceedings 36 (2004): 1920–21, reviewed in G. Switzer, M. A. Dew, and R. Twillman, "Psychosocial Issues in Living Organ Donation," in *The Transplant Patient: Biological, Psychiatric and Ethical Issues in Organ Transplantation*, ed. P. Trzepacz and A. Dimartini (Cambridge: Cambridge University Press, 2000); and K. K. Clemens, H. Thiessen-Philbrook, et al., "Psychosocial Health of Living Kidney Donors," *American Journal of Transplantation* 6 (2006): 2965–77.

40. Schover, Streem, et al., "The Psychosocial Impact of Donating a Kidney; J. Hiller, M. Sroka, et al., "Identifying Donor Concerns to Increase Live Organ Donation," *Journal of Transplant Coordination* 8 (1998): 51–54; M. Andersen, L. Mathisen, et al., "Living Donors' Experiences One Week after Donating a Kidney," *Clinical Transplantation* 19 (2005): 90–96.

41. Johnson, Anderson, et al., "Long-Term Follow-Up of Living Kidney Donors"; Hiller, Sroka, et al., "Identifying Donor Concerns."

42. Johnson, Anderson, et al., "Long-Term Follow-Up of Living Kidney Donors"; Schover, Streem, et al., "The Psychosocial Impact of Donating a Kidney"; M. Smith, D. Kappell, et al., "Living-Related Kidney Donors: A Multi-Center Study of Donor Education, Socioeconomic Adjustment, and Rehabilitation," *American Journal of Kidney Diseases* 8 (1986): 223–33.

43. Johnson, Anderson, et al., "Long-Term Follow-Up of Living Kidney Donors"; Smith, Kappell, et al., "Living-Related Kidney Donors"; C. Jacobs, E. Johnson, et al., "Kidney Transplants from Living Donors: How Donation Affects Family Dynamics," *Advances in Renal Replacement Therapy* 5 (1998): 89–97.

44. Schover, Streem, et al., "The Psychosocial Impact of Donating a Kidney"; Jacobs, Johnson, et al., "Kidney Transplants from Living Donors"; T. Peters, S. Repper, et al., "Living Kidney Donation: Recovery and Return to Activities of Daily Living," *Clinical Transplantation* 14 (2000): 433–38.

45. Virginia Postrel, donor to Sally Satel, personal communication with Satel, August 15, 2008.

Chapter 2: The Cost-Effectiveness of Renal Transplantation

1. R. Klar, "Cost-Treatment of Chronic Renal Disease," memorandum to assistant secretary for health, Department of Health, Education, and Welfare, 1972, as cited in Paul W. Eggers, "Medicare's End Stage Renal Disease Program," *Health Care Financing Review* 22, no. 1 (Fall 2000): 55–60.

2. Ibid., 57.

3. U.S. Renal Data System, *USRDS 2007 Annual Data Report: Atlas of Chronic Kidney Disease and End-Stage Renal Disease in the United States*, 2007, table D.4, http://www.usrds.org/2007/view/4_d.html (accessed January 8, 2008).

4. The figure of $229 million is from Richard A. Rettig, "The Federal Government and Social Planning for End-Stage Renal Disease: Past, Present, and Future," *Seminars in*

Nephrology 2 (1982): 111; the figure of $250 million is from Eggers, "Medicare's End Stage Renal Disease Program," 58.

5. Paul W. Eggers, "A Quarter Century of Medicare Expenditures for End Stage Renal Disease," *Seminars in Nephrology* 20, no. 6 (November 2000): 516–19.

6. U.S. Renal Data System, *USRDS 2007 Annual Data Report*, figure 11.7, http://www.usrds.org/2007/view/11_econ.asp (accessed January 8, 2008).

7. Jay L. Xue, Jennie Z. Ma, Thomas A. Louis, and Allan J. Collins, "Forecast of the Number of Patients with End-Stage Renal Disease in the United States to the Year 2010," *Journal of the American Society of Nephrology* 12, no. 12 (2001): 2757. Of all hemodialysis patients, close to 42 percent were covered solely by Medicare in 2005, while 33.7 percent were under Medicare/Medicaid. Slightly more than 90 percent in all had some type of Medicare coverage. U.S. Renal Data System, *USRDS 2007 Annual Data Report*, figure 4.5, http://www.usrds.org/2007/view/04_modalities.asp (accessed January 8, 2008).

8. U.S. Renal Data System, USRDS 2007 Annual Data Report, précis, http://www.usrds.org/2007/pdf/00a_precis_07.pdf (accessed April 3, 2008).

9. Eggers, "Medicare's End Stage Renal Disease Program," 58.

10. Jesse D. Schold, Titte R. Srinivas, Liise K. Kayler, and Herwig-Ulf Meier-Kriesche, "The Overlapping Risk Profile between Dialysis Patients Listed and Not Listed for Renal Transplantation," *American Journal of Transplantation* 8, no. 1 (2008): 58–68.

11. U.S. Renal Data System, *USRDS 2007 Annual Data Report*, 236, table H.31, http://www.usrds.org/2007/ref/H_morte_07.pdf (accessed January 8, 2008).

12. Paul L. Kimmel and Samir S. Patel, "Quality of Life in Patients with Chronic Kidney Disease: Focus on End-Stage Renal Disease Treated with Hemodialysis," *Seminars in Nephrology* 26, no. 1 (2006): 68–79.

13. M. R. Gold, J. E. Siegel, L. B. Russell, and M. C. Weinstein, *Cost-Effectiveness in Health and Medicine* (Oxford: Oxford University Press, 1996).

14. M. F. Drummond, B. J. O'Brien, G. L. Stoddart, and G. W. Torrance (eds.), "Cost-Benefit Analysis," in *Methods for the Economic Evaluation of Health Care Programmes*, 2d ed., 205–11 (Oxford: Oxford University Press, 1999).

15. L. B. Russell, M. R. Gold, J. E. Siegel, N. Daniels, and M. C. Weinstein, "The Role of Cost-Effectiveness Analysis in Health and Medicine," *Journal of the American Medical Association* 276, no. 15 (1996): 1253–58.

16. D. Meltzer, "Accounting for Future Costs in Medical Cost-Effectiveness Analysis," *Journal of Health Economics* 16, no. 1 (1997): 33–64.

17. P. J. Neumann, S. J. Goldie, and M. C. Weinstein, "Preference-Based Measures in Economic Evaluation in Health Care," *Annual Review of Public Health* 21 (2000): 587–611.

18. C. J. Murray, "Quantifying the Burden of Disease: The Technical Basis for Disability-Adjusted Life Years," *Bulletin of the World Health Organization* 72, no. 3 (1994): 429–45.

19. W. C. Winkelmayer, M. C. Weinstein, M. A. Mittleman, R. J. Glynn, and J. S. Pliskin, "Health Economic Evaluations: The Special Case of End-Stage Renal Disease Treatment," *Medical Decision Making* 22, no. 5 (2002): 417–30.

20. R. A. Hirth, M. E. Chernew, E. Miller, A. M. Fendrick, and W. G. Weissert, "Willingness to Pay for Quality-Adjusted Life Year: In Search of a Standard," *Medical Decision Making* 20, no. 3 (2000): 332–42.

21. Winkelmayer et al., "Health Economic Evaluations."

22. H. E. Klarman, J. O. S. Francis, and G. D. Rosenthal, "Cost Effectiveness Analysis Applied to the Treatment of Chronic Renal Disease," *Medical Care* 6, no. 1 (1968): 48–54; P. V. Stange and A. T. Sumner, "Predicting Treatment Costs and Life Expectancy for End-Stage Renal Disease," *New England Journal of Medicine* 298, no. 7 (1978): 372–78; S. D. Roberts, D. R. Maxwell, and T. L. Gross, "Cost-Effective Care of End-Stage Renal Disease: A Billion Dollar Question," *Annals of Internal Medicine* 92, no. 2, pt. 1 (1980): 243–48; A. Ludbrook, "A Cost-Effectiveness Analysis of the Treatment of Chronic Renal Failure," *Applied Economics* 13, no. 3 (1981): 337–50; T. Schersten, H. Brynger, I. Karlberg, and E. Jonsson, "Cost-Effectiveness Analysis of Organ Transplantation," *International Journal of Technology Assessment in Health Care* 2, no. 3 (1986): 545–52; T. I. Garner and R. Dardis, "Cost-Effectiveness Analysis of End-Stage Renal Disease Treatments," *Medical Care* 25, no. 1 (1987): 25–34; R. Sesso, J. M. Eisenberg, C. Stabile, S. Draibe, H. Azjen, and O. Ramos, "Cost-Effectiveness Analysis of the Treatment of End-Stage Renal Disease in Brazil," *International Journal of Technology Assessment in Health Care* 6, no. 1 (1990): 107–14; B. E. Croxson and T. Ashton, "A Cost-Effectiveness Analysis of the Treatment of End Stage Renal Failure," *New Zealand Medical Journal* 103, no. 888 (1990): 171–74; I. Karlberg and G. Nyberg, "Cost-Effectiveness Analysis of Renal Transplantation," *International Journal of Technology Assessment in Health Care* 11, no. 2 (1995): 611–22; A. Laupacis, P. Keown, N. Pus, H. Krueger, B. Ferguson, C. Wong, and N. Muirhead, "A Study of the Quality of Life and Cost-Utility of Renal Transplantation," *Kidney International* 50, no. 1 (1996): 235–42; G. A. de Wit, P. G. Ramsteijn, and F. T. de Charro, "Economic Evaluation of End Stage Renal Disease Treatment," *Health Policy* 44, no. 3 (1998): 215–32; M. Kaminota, "Cost-Effectiveness Analysis of Dialysis and Kidney Transplantation in Japan," *Keio Journal of Medicine* 50, no. 2 (2001): 100–108; S. V. Jassal, M. D. Krahn, G. Naglie, J. S. Zaltzman, J. M. Roscoe, E. H. Cole, and D. A. Redelmeier, "Kidney Transplantation in the Elderly: A Decision Analysis," *Journal of the American Society of Nephrology* 14, no. 1 (2003): 187–96; J. F. Whiting, B. Kiberd, Z. Kalo, P. Keown, L. Roels, and M. Kjerulf, "Cost-Effectiveness of Organ Donation: Evaluating Investment in Donor Action and Other Donor Initiatives," *American Journal of Transplantation* 4 (2004): 569–73; Arthur J. Matas and Mark A. Schnitzler, "Payment for Living Donor (Vendor) Kidneys: A Cost-Effectiveness Analysis," *American Journal of Transplantation* 4 (2003): 216–21; I. Cleemput, K. Kesteloot, Y. Vanrenterghem, and S. De Geest, "The Economic Implications of Non-adherence after Renal Transplantation," *Pharmacoeconomics* 22, no. 18 (2004): 1217–34; J. C. Hornberger, J. H. Best, and L. P. Garrison Jr., "Cost-Effectiveness of Repeat Medical Procedures: Kidney Transplantation as an Example," *Medical Decision Making* 17, no. 4 (1997): 363–72.

23. Klarman et al., "Cost Effectiveness Analysis Applied to the Treatment of Chronic Renal Disease."

24. Cleemput et al., "The Economic Implications of Non-adherence after Renal Transplantation."

25. Jassal et al., "Kidney Transplantation in the Elderly."

26. E. S. Huang, L. Jin, M. Shook, M. H. Chin, D. O. Meltzer, "The Impact of Patient Preferences on the Cost-Effectiveness of Intensive Glucose Control in Older Patients with New Onset Diabetes," *Diabetes Care* 29, no. 2 (2006): 259–64.

27. Hornberger et al., "Cost-Effectiveness of Repeat Medical Procedures."

28. Matas and Schnitzler, "Payment for Living Donor (Vendor) Kidneys." An alternative way to determine the monetary value of a kidney is to estimate how much compensation is required before an individual is indifferent to selling a kidney or not. A study by Becker and Elías estimated this value by calculating the dollar amount required to balance the three major risks or harms associated with selling a kidney: risk of death, risk of reduced quality of life, and time lost during recovery. Using this method, the study valued a kidney at $15,200. Gary S. Becker and Julio Elías, "Introducing Incentives in the Market for Live and Cadaveric Organ Donations," *Journal of Economic Perspectives* 21, no. 3 (2006): 3–24.

29. Matas and Schnitzler, "Payment for Living Donor (Vendor) Kidneys."

30. X. Su, S. A. Zenios, and G. M. Chertow, "Incorporating Recipient Choice in Kidney Transplantation," *Journal of the American Society of Nephrology* 15 (2004): 1656–63.

Chapter 3: Operational Organization of a System for Compensated Living Organ Providers

1. As part of the U.S. Department of Health and Human Service's Gift of Life Donation Initiative, the HRSA launched in April 2003 the "Organ Donation Breakthrough Collaborative" to identify and promote best practices in organ donation for adoption by hospitals and organ procurement organizations (see http://www.unos.org/news/news Detail.asp?id=307); W. H. Marks, D. Wagner, T. C. Pearson, J. P. Orlowski, P. W. Nelson, J. J. McGowan, M. K. Guidinger, and J. Burdick, "Organ Donation and Utilization, 1995–2004: Entering the Collaborative Era," *American Journal of Transplantation* 5, no. 2 (2006): 1101–10; T. J. Shafer, D. Wagner, J. Chessare, F. A. Zampiello, V. McBride, and J. Perdue, "Organ donation breakthrough collaborative: increasing organ donation through system redesign," *Critical Care Nurse* 26, no. 2 (April 2006): 33–42, 44–8; quiz 49.

2. Alvin E. Roth, Tayfun Sonmez, M. Utku Unver, Francis L. Delmonico, and Susan L. Saidman, "Utilizing List Exchange and Nondirected Donation Through 'Chain' Paired Kidney Donations," *American Journal of Transplantation* 6, no. 11 (November 2006): 2694–2705.

3. U.S. House of Representatives, Committee on Energy and Commerce, Subcommittee on Oversight and Investigations, *Assessing Initiatives to Increase Organ Donations: Hearing Before the Subcommittee on Oversight and Investigations of the House*

Committee on Energy and Commerce, 108th Cong., 1st sess., June 3, 2003, statement of Robert M. Sade, professor of surgery, Medical University of South Carolina, http://energycommerce.house.gov/reparchives/108/Hearings/06032003hearing946/print.htm (accessed March 12, 2008).

4. Ellen Sheehy, Suzanne L. Conrad, Lori E. Brigham, Richard Luskin, Phyllis Weber, Mark Eakin, Lawrence Schkade, and Lawrence Hunsicker, "Estimating the Number of Potential Organ Donors in the United States," *New England Journal of Medicine* 349, no. 7 (August 2007): 667–74.

5. We have specifically chosen to refer to persons being financially compensated for the provision of kidneys as *compensated providers* rather than donors. The distinction separates the act of *donating* an organ (still permissible under our new proposal) from receiving compensation for undergoing surgical removal of a kidney for the purpose of *providing* a kidney for transplantation. In most other contexts, including the other chapters in this book, people providing organs continue to be referred to as donors, whether compensated or not.

6. Organ Procurement and Transplantation Network and the Scientific Registry of Transplant Recipients, *2006 OPTN/SRTR Annual Report,* figure 4-5 and tables 5.14 a, b, and c.

7. Under the current system, when a deceased-donor organ becomes available, a computerized algorithm developed by the Organ Procurement and Transplant Network and UNOS and approved by the OPTN board is used to identify a potential recipient. The algorithm allocates standard deceased-donor kidneys on a point system. Points are awarded to listed candidates based on blood type, waiting time, quality of antigen (tissue) match, level of sensitization, and whether or not the candidate is a child. The allocation is further defined within specific geographic regions. See United Network for Organ Sharing, "Definition of Expanded Criteria Donor and Standard Donor," in *The Point System for Kidney Allocation,* policy 3.5.11, June 20, 2008, http://www.unos.org/PoliciesandBylaws2/policies/docs/policy_7.doc (accessed August 1, 2008).

8. See chapter 8 for an argument that the states, rather than the federal government, would be the most appropriate loci of control of a donor compensation program.

9. Association of Organ Procurement Organizations, "AOPO Accredited OPOs, Effective September 1, 2007," http://www.aopo.org/aopo/content/doc/Accredited OPOs-alpha9-7-07.pdf (accessed March 7, 2008).

10. Association of Organ Procurement Organizations, "Our Mission," http://www.aopo.org/aopo/index.asp (accessed March 7, 2008).

11. United Network for Organ Sharing, "Definition of Expanded Criteria Donor and Standard Donor," http://www.unos.org/PoliciesandBylaws2/policies/docs/policy_7.doc.

12. See note 7, above.

13. As designated by the human leukocyte antigen (HLA) system. HLA proteins on the outer part of body cells are unique to each person. These proteins are used for "matching" between donor and recipient in transplantation.

14. Health Insurance Portability and Accountability Act 1996. Public Law 104–191.

15. Such a regionally based mechanism could be employed if states or geographic regions, rather than the federal government, were directing the compensation scheme.

16. These criteria comprise a comprehensive list of tests and evaluations which address a widely diverse group of potential living donors. The compensated-provider program would likely require a more focused evaluation if the eligibility criteria were sufficiently strict to exclude older providers and/or providers with significant medical illnesses. For example, restriction to individuals between the ages of thirty and forty-five without diabetes, hypertension, or obesity would most likely make colonoscopy or invasive cardiac evaluation unnecessary.

17. Mary A. Dew, Cheryl L. Jacobs, Sheila G. Jowsey, Ruthanne Hanto, Charles Miller, and Francis L. Delmonico, "United Network for Organ Sharing, American Society of Transplant Surgeons, American Society of Transplantation Meeting Notes: Guidelines for the Psychosocial Evaluation of Living Unrelated Kidney Donors in the United States," *American Journal of Transplantation* 7, no. 5 (May 2007): 1047–54; Organ Procurement and Transplantation Network and United Network for Organ Sharing, "Living Kidney Donor Evaluation Guidelines," http://www.unos.org/ContentDocuments/Living_ Kidney_Donor_Evaluation_Guidelines2(1).pdf (accessed March 7, 2008).

18. United Network for Organ Sharing, "Allocation of Deceased Kidneys," in Resources: Policies, section 3.5, December 18, 2007, http://www.unos.org/Policiesand Bylaws2/policies/pdfs/policy_7.pdf (accessed March 7, 2008).

19. As we explain later, all the costs related to the provider, including those for travel and required weeks of stay, would be covered by the OPO and thus factored into the price charged to the transplant center.

20. Note that the price of the organ charged to the transplant centers is going to be more than the financial compensation for providers, since OPOs have other costs (such as donor screening and administrative costs).

21. Arthur Matas, "A Gift of Life Deserves Compensation: How to Increase Living Kidney Donation with Realistic Incentives," Cato Institute Policy Analysis No. 604 (November 7, 2007).

22. See chapters 4, 5, and 6.

23. Gary S. Becker and Julio J. Elías, "Introducing Incentives in the Market for Live and Cadaveric Organ Donations," *Journal of Economic Perspectives* 21, no. 3 (Summer 2007): 3–24. Arthur J. Matas and Mark A. Schnitzler, "Payment for Living Donor (Vendor) Kidneys: A Cost-Effectiveness Analysis," *American Journal of Transplantation* 4, no. 2 (February 2004): 216–21.

24. See chapter 2.

25. If the screening is strict and the providers healthy, two years is reasonable and fair. Because organ providers would be an exceptionally healthy group, such coverage, from an actuarial standpoint, should be inexpensive. This is consistent with recommendations put forth by others; see, for example, Matas, "A Gift of Life Deserves Compensation," and Robert S. Gaston, Gabriel M. Danovitch, Richard A. Epstein, Jeffery P. Kahn, Arthur J. Matas, and Mark A. Schnitzler, "Limiting Financial Disincentives in Live Organ

Donation: A Rational Solution to the Kidney Shortage," *American Journal of Transplantation* 6, no. 11 (November 2006): 2548–55.

26. Organ Procurement and Transplantation Network and the Scientific Registry of Transplant Recipients, *2007 OPTN/SRTR Annual Report*. Chapter IV, figure IV-6, 7 and table IV-3

27. See chapter 2.

Chapter 4: Donor Compensation without Exploitation

1. Debra Saunders, "American Vampire," *San Francisco Chronicle*, April 25, 2006.

2. Richard Morais, "Desperate Arrangements," *Forbes*, January 29, 2007; John Cornwell, "The Body Shops," *Sunday Times* (London), March 25, 2007.

3. See M. Goyal, R. Mehta, L. Schneiderman, and A. Sehgal, "Economic and Health Consequences of Selling a Kidney in India," *Journal of the American Medical Association* 288 (2002): 1589–92.

4. David Matas and David Kilgour, *An Independent Investigation into Allegations of Organ Harvesting of Falun Gong Practitioners in China*, January 31, 2007, http://organharvestinvestigation.net (accessed December 9, 2007).

5. William Plant, "Is It Desirable to Legitimize Paid Living Donor Kidney Transplantation Programmes? Evidence Against," in *Living Donor Kidney Transplantation*, ed. Robert Gaston and Jonas Wadstrom, 180–90 (London: Taylor and Francis, 2005).

6. Garwood, "Dilemma Over Live-Donor Transplantation."

7. Steering Committee of the Istanbul Summit, "Organ Trafficking and Transplant Tourism and Commercialism: The Declaration of Istanbul," *Lancet* 372 (July 5, 2008): 5.

8. As of early 2008, De Leon remains healthy and employed in construction work; see National Geographic Channel, "Inside the Body Trade," *Explorer*, November 5, 2007.

9. Ibid.

10. Transplantation Society, "Policy and Ethics," http://www.transplantation-soc.org/policy.php (accessed October 27, 2007).

11. Gabriel M. Danovitch and Alan B. Leichtman, "Kidney Vending: The 'Trojan Horse' of Organ Transplantation," *Clinical Journal of the American Society of Nephrology* 1 (October 2006): 1133–35.

12. George Abouna, M. M. Sabawi, M. S. A. Kumar, and M. Samhan, "The Negative Impact of Paid Organ Donation," in *Organ Replacement Therapy: Ethics, Justice, Commerce*, ed. Walter Land and John Dossetor, 164–72 (New York: Springer-Verlag, 1991), 169. See also chapters 5 and 7, below.

13. Notably, however, bills to prohibit organ trading have been proposed in the Pakistani government at regular intervals since 1992.

14. Technically, this is different from a so-called "gray market," which typically refers to the passage of goods through unauthorized distribution channels when authorized

channels exist. In a gray market, consumers who inadvertently buy from unauthorized sellers may be protected by the law. In Pakistan, no channels are authorized; there is no protection against fraudulent or defective goods purchased in gray markets. See Fakhar Rehman and Carol Grisanti, "Pakistan's Kidney Bazaar," *MSNBC World Blog*, September 5, 2007, http://worldblog.msnbc.msn.com/archive/2007/09/05/345490.aspx (accessed January 4, 2008).

15. Morais, "Desperate Arrangements."

16. Katrina A. Bramstedt and Jun Xu, "Checklist: Passport, Plane Ticket, Organ Transplant," *American Journal of Transplantation* 7, no. 7 (July 2007): 1698–1701.

17. Robert Gaston, MD, personal conversation with the author, November 19, 2007.

18. Interestingly, one of the most vocal supporters of legal, regulated markets in India, K. C. Reddy, does, indeed, inform his prospective donors of the risks that they run. See K. C. Reddy, "Should Paid Organ Donation Be Banned in India? To Buy or Let Die?" *National Medical Journal of India* 6 (1993): 137–39.

19. Pat Sidley, "News Roundup: South African Doctors Charged with Involvement in Organ Trade," *British Medical Journal* 329, no. 7459 (July 24, 2004): 190.

20. Laura Meckler, "Kidney Shortage Inspires a Radical Idea: Organ Sales," *Wall Street Journal*, November 13, 2007.

21. Vivekanand Jha and Kirpal S. Chugh, "The Case Against a Regulated System of Living Kidney Sales," *Nature Clinical Practice Nephrology* 2 (2006): 466–67.

22. U.S. House of Representatives, Committee on Energy and Commerce, Subcommittee on Oversight and Investigation, *Assessing Initiatives to Increase Organ Donations: Hearing Before the Subcommittee on Oversight and Investigations, of the Committee on Energy and Commerce*, 108th Cong., 1st sess., June 3, 2003, 67.

23. Nancy Scheper-Hughes, "Rotten Trade: Millennial Capitalism, Human Values and Global Justice in Organs Trafficking," *Journal of Human Rights* 2, no. 2 (2003): 197–226; Nancy Scheper-Hughes, "The Ultimate Commodity," *Lancet* 366 (2005): 1349–50; Vivekanand Jha, "Paid Transplants in India: The Grim Reality," *Nephrology, Dialysis, and Transplantation* 19, no. 3 (2004): 541–43.

24. See James Stacey Taylor, "A 'Queen of Hearts' Trial of Organ Markets? Why Scheper-Hughes's Objections to Markets in Human Organs Fail," *Journal of Medical Ethics* 33 (2007): 201–4.

25. James Stacey Taylor, "Why the 'Black Market' Arguments against Legalizing Organ Sales Fail," *Res Publica* 12, no. 2 (June 2006): 163–78; James Stacey Taylor, *Stakes and Kidneys: Why Markets in Human Body Parts are Morally Imperative* (Aldershot, UK: Ashgate, 2005), 173–81.

26. Taylor, "Why the 'Black Market' Arguments against Legalizing Organ Sales Fail."

27. See A. Matas, "The Case for Living Kidney Sales: Rationale, Objections and Concerns," *American Journal of Transplantation* 4 (2004): 2007–17.

28. As Benjamin Hippen has argued, any defensible compensation scheme for human organs would have to meet four conditions: It would have to be safe for both the donor

and the recipient; it would have to be transparent; each participating institution would have to state its position regarding such compensation; and it would have to be subject to the rule of law. Benjamin Hippen, "In Defense of a Regulated Market in Kidneys from Living Vendors," *Journal of Medicine and Philosophy* 30 (2005): 593–626.

29. Ibid., 175.

30. Goyal et al., "Economic and Health Consequences of Selling a Kidney in India."

31. See, for example, Deborah Josefson, "Selling a Kidney Fails to Rescue Indians from Poverty," *British Medical Journal* 325 (2002): 795.

32. An authoritative 1997 report warned that the Transplantation of Human Organs Act had merely pushed the country to the center of "an even larger underground market controlled and organised by cash-rich crime gangs expanding out from the heroin trade into the organs trade." See Rashmee Ahmed, "UK Doctor Puts Indian Kidneys Up for Sale," *Times of India*, August 28, 2002, http://timesofindia.indiatimes.com/articleshow/20479282.cms (accessed December 20, 2007), and Ganapati Mudur, "Indian Doctors Debate Incentives for Organ Donors," *British Medical Journal* 329 (2004): 938.

33. Goyal et al., "Economic and Health Consequences of Selling a Kidney in India," 1591.

34. Jeffrey P. Kahn, "Studying Organ Sales: Short Term Profits, Long Term Suffering," *CNN Online*, October 10, 2002, http://archives.cnn.com/2002/HEALTH/10/01/ethics.matters.selling.organs (accessed November 5, 2007).

35. Francis L. Delmonico, Robert Arnold, Nancy Scheper-Hughes, Laura A. Siminoff Jeffrey Kahn, and Stuart J. Youngner, "Ethical Incentives—Not Payment—For Organ Donation," *New England Journal of Medicine* 346, no. 25 (June 2002): 2004.

36. *Stanford Encyclopedia of Philosophy*, s.v. "Coercion," http://plato.stanford.edu/entries/coercion (accessed November 19, 2007).

37. Ezekiel Jonathan Emanuel, "Undue Inducement: Nonsense on Stilts?" *American Journal of Bioethics* 5, no. 5 (2005): 9–13.

38. James Stacey Taylor, "Autonomy, Inducements, and Organ Sales," in *Philosophical Reflections on Medical Ethics*, ed. Nafsika Athanassoulis, 135–59 (London: Palgrave McMillan, 2006).

39. Virgina Postrel, "Organ Donation Incentives," *Dynamist.com*, http://www.dynamist.com/weblog/archives/002168.html (accessed November 5, 2007).

40. J. Radcliffe Richards, A. S. Daar, R. D. Guttmann, R. Hoffenberg, I. Kennedy, M. Lock, R. A. Sells, and N. Tilney, "The Case for Allowing Kidney Sales," *Lancet* 351 (1998): 1950–52.

41. Danovitch and Leichtman, "Kidney Vending."

42. For more on how such safeguards might work in a compensated donor system, see chapter 3.

43. Nancy Scheper-Hughes, "The Ends of the Body: Commodity Fetishism and the Global Traffic in Organs," *SAIS Review of International Affairs* 22, no. 1 (Winter–Spring 2002): 61–80.

44. Sam Vaknin, "Organ Trafficking in Eastern Europe," *American Chronicle*, September 7, 2007, http://www.americanchronicle.com/articles/viewArticle.asp?articleID= 37057 (accessed December 20, 2007).

45. Rick Weiss, "A Look at . . . the Body Shop: At the Heart of an Uneasy Commerce," *Washington Post*, June 27, 1999.

46. UNOS to Sally Satel, MD, November 24, 2006. As of October 31, 2006, 18.5 percent of adult registrants said they were "working for income" when first listed by UNOS (35.2 percent did not respond to this question). Thus, even if we assume that all nonrespondents were, in fact, working for income, 53.7 percent would be the upper limit of those working for a living. With respect to education, 6.2 percent said their "highest education level at listing" was grade school, while 39.3 percent said high school. Only 11 percent had associate or bachelor level degrees.

47. BBC2, "Iran Kidney Sale," *This World*, October 31, 2006, http://news.bbc.co.uk/ 2/hi/programmes/this_world/6080328.stm (accessed January 4, 2008).

48. Muna T. Canales, Bertram L. Kasiske, and Mark E. Rosenberg, "Transplantation Tourism: Outcomes of United States Residents Who Undergo Kidney Transplantation Overseas," *Transplantation* 81, no. 12 (2006): 1658–61; Living Non-Related Renal Transplant Study Group, "Commercially Motivated Renal Transplantation: Results in 540 People Transplanted in India," *Clinical Transplantation* 11, no. 6 (1997): 536–44; Sean E. Kennedy, Yvonne Shen, John A. Charlesworth, James D. Mackie, John D. Mahony, John J. P. Kelly, and Bruce A. Pussell, "Outcome of Overseas Commercial Kidney Transplantation: An Australian Perspective," *Medical Journal of Australia* 182, no. 5 (2005): 224–27; Mehmet Sükrü Sever, Rümeyza Kazancioglu, Alaattin Yildiz, Aydin Türkmen, Tevfik Ecder, S. Mehmet Kayacan, Vedat Çelik, Sevgi Sahin, A. Emin Aydin, Ulug Eldegez, and Ergin Ark, "Outcome of Living Unrelated (Commercial) Renal Transplantation," *Kidney International* 60 (2001): 1477–83; Nicholas G. Inston, D. Gill, A. Al-Hakim, and Andrew Ready, "Living Paid Organ Transplantation Results in Unacceptably High Recipient Morbidity and Mortality," *Transplantation Proceedings* 37, no. 2 (March 2005): 560–62.

49. Mark J. Cherry, "Is a Market for Human Organs Necessarily Exploitative?" *Public Affairs Quarterly* 14, no. 4 (2000): 341.

50. Ahad J. Ghods and S. Shekoufeh, "Iranian Model of Paid and Regulated Living Unrelated Kidney Donation," *Clinical Journal of the American Society of Nephrology* 1 (2006): 1136–45.

51. Shahrzad Ossareh, Masoomeh Asl, Shams Al-Zubairi, and Soubia Naseem, "Attitude of Iranian Nephrologists toward Living Unrelated Kidney Donation," *Transplantation Proceedings* 39, no. 4 (May 2007): 819–21.

52. As noted by Ahad J. Ghods, S. Savaj, and P. Khosravani, "Adverse Effects of a Controlled Living-Unrelated Donor Renal Transplant Program on Living-Related and Cadaveric Kidney Donation," *Transplantation Proceedings* 32, no. 3 (May 2000): 541.

53. Benjamin E. Hippen, "Organ Sales and Moral Travails: Lessons from the Living Kidney Vendor Program in Iran," *Cato Policy Study*, Cato Institute, March 2008. The

Iranian system provides an example of how markets and altruism can coexist, if given the chance. Since 2000, Iran has had in place a system for donation of cadaveric organs. (The reason it did not have one sooner is that the Iranian parliament did not recognize brain death as death.) This program is steadily growing, with the number of cadaveric organs donated having risen tenfold in six years from approximately 20 kidneys in 2000 to about 230 in 2006. This increase in cadaveric donation has occurred during a time at which the number of paid organ donors has stayed about the same. As such, then, it is clear that the altruistic donation of organs will still occur even if a system of compensated donation is in place. Also from Benjamin Hippen, MD, personal conversation with the author, December 10, 2007.

54. Parvathi Menon, Asha Krishnakumar, V. Sridhar, Ravi Sharma, and Lyla Bavadam, "Kidneys Still for Sale," *Hindu* 14, no. 25 (December 1997), http://www.hinduonnet.com/fline/fl1425/14250640.htm (accessed January 4, 2008). The question of "crowding out" is covered in greater depth in chapters 5 and 7, below.

55. Benjamin Hippen, "The Case for Kidney Markets," *New Atlantis*, no. 14 (Fall 2006): 47–61.

Chapter 5: Concerns about Human Dignity and Commodification

1. Barbara Feder Ostrov, "Transplant Dilemma Grows," *San Jose Mercury News*, November 26, 2006.

2. Ibid.

3. The program closed in May 2006 following revelations of administrative irregularities; see Victoria Colliver, "Kaiser Kidney Transplant Unit to Close Down," *San Francisco Chronicle*, May 13, 2006, http://www.sfgate.com/cgi-bin/article.cgi?f=/c/a/2006/05/13/KAISER.TMP (accessed May 30, 2008).

4. Laura Meckler, "Why It's Hard to Give Away a Kidney," *Wall Street Journal*, December 26, 2007, D1.

5. Section 301 of the 1984 National Organ Transplant Act imposes criminal penalties of up to $50,000 and five years in prison on any person who "knowingly acquire[s], receive[s], or otherwise transfer[s] any human organ for valuable consideration for use in human transplantation if the transfer affects interstate commerce." See appendix A and chapter 8, below, for further information and discussion.

6. Francis L. Delmonico, Robert Arnold, Nancy Scheper-Hughes, Laura A. Siminoff Jeffrey Kahn, and Stuart J. Youngner, "Ethical Incentives—Not Payment—For Organ Donation," *New England Journal of Medicine* 346, no. 25 (June 2002): 2004.

7. U.S. House of Representatives, Committee on Energy and Commerce, Subcommittee on Oversight and Investigations, *Assessing Initiatives to Increase Organ Donations: Hearing Before the Subcommittee on Oversight and Investigations of the House Committee on Energy and Commerce*, 108th Cong., 1st sess. (June 3, 2003), statement of Francis L. Delmonico, 66.

8. Cynthia B. Cohen, "Public Policy and the Sale of Human Organs," *Kennedy Institute of Ethics Journal* 12, no. 1 (March 2002): 48.

9. Leon R. Kass, "The Wisdom of Repugnance," *New Republic* 216, no. 22 (June 2, 1997): 17–26.

10. Steven Pinker, "The Stupidity of Dignity," *New Republic*, May 28, 2008, http://www.tnr.com/story_print.html?id=d8731cf4-e87b-4d88-b7e7-f5059cd0bfbd (accessed June 5, 2008).

11. Ruth Macklin, "Human Dignity is a Useless Concept," *British Medical Journal* 327, no. 7429 (December 20, 2003): 1419–20, http://www.bmj.com/cgi/content/full/327/7429/1419 (accessed June 5, 2008).

12. Michael J. Sandel, "What Money Can't Buy: The Moral Limits of Markets," *Tanner Lectures on Human Values* (Brasenose College, Oxford, May 11–12, 1998), 93, http://www.tannerlectures.utah.edu/lectures/documents/sandel00.pdf (accessed April 9, 2008).

13. Alvin E. Roth, "Repugnance as a Constraint on Markets," *Journal of Economic Perspectives* 21, no. 3 (Summer 2007): 37–58; Marion Fourcade and Kieran Healy, "Moral Views of a Market Society," *Annual Review of Sociology* 33 (August 2007): 105–128.

14. Martha C. Nussbaum, "'Whether from Reason or Prejudice': Taking Money For Bodily Services," *Journal of Legal Studies* 27, no. 2 (June 1998): 693–724.

15. Adam Smith, *An Inquiry Into the Nature and Causes of the Wealth of Nations* (London: T. Nelson and Sons, 1895), 44.

16. Nussbaum, "'Whether from Reason or Prejudice,'" 693.

17. Viviana Zelizer, "Human Values and the Market: The Case of Life Insurance and Death in 19th-Century America," *American Journal of Sociology* 84, no. 3 (November 1978): 591.

18. Code of Hammurabi, http://www.wsu.edu/~dee/MESO/CODE.HTM (accessed December 27, 2007).

19. Pinker, "Stupidity of Dignity."

20. See Robert Arnold, Steven Bartlett, James Bernat, John Colonna, Donald Dafoe, Nancy Dubler, Scott Gruber, Jeffrey Kahn, Richard Luskin, Howard Nathan, Susan Orloff, Jeffrey Prottas, Robyn Shapiro, Camillo Ricordi, Stuart Youngner, and Francis L. Delmonico, "Financial Incentives for Cadaver Donation: An Ethical Reappraisal," *Transplantation* 73, no. 8 (April 2002): 1361. On the other hand, the members deem it ethically permissible for the transplant community to "convey appreciation" to the families of deceased organ donors by reimbursing funeral expenses or making charitable contributions in the names of the deceased. This is a curious decision, because payment of funeral expenses could surely serve as an incentive to donate, irrespective of whether it is intended as a "thank you."

21. John Paul II, "Address of the Holy Father John Paul II to the 18th International Congress of the Transplantation Society," Rome, August 29, 2000, http://www.vatican.va/holy_father/john_paul_ii/speeches/2000/jul-sep/documents/hf_jp-ii_spe_20000829_transplants_en.html (accessed December 26, 2007).

22. Stephen Wilkinson, *Bodies for Sale—Ethics and Exploitation in the Human Body Trade* (London: Routledge, 2003), 46.

23. Margaret Jane Radin, *Contested Commodities* (Boston, Mass.: Harvard University Press, 1996), 114.

24. The author is grateful to Jonathan Moreno, who is the David and Lyn Silfen University Professor and professor of medical ethics and of history and sociology of science at the University of Pennsylvania, for this insight (and the Yiddish). Personal communication, July 2, 2008.

25. Sandel, "What Money Can't Buy," 94.

26. Jay Baruch, "Prisoners and Organ Donation," *Medicine & Health Rhode Island* 88, no. 12 (December 2005): 438, http://www.rimed.org/pdf/mhri/m05Decmhri.pdf (accessed January 31, 2008).

27. James F. Childress and Catharyn T. Liverman, eds., *Organ Donation: Opportunities for Action* (Washington, D.C.: National Academies Press, 2006), 80.

28. See subsequent discussion in chapter 5.

29. Observed by the author in a District of Columbia Metro train station, September 2007. See also www.123donate.com.

30. Gabrielle Glaser, "Oregon Births a Boom in Surrogate Babies," *Oregonian*, July 9, 2006.

31. Javaad Zargooshi, "Quality of Life of Iranian Kidney 'Donors,'" *Journal of Urology* 166, no. 5 (November 2001): 1790–99; Javaad Zargooshi, "Iranian Kidney Donors: Motivations and Relations with Recipients," *Journal of Urology* 165, no. 2 (February 2001): 386–92.

32. Lori B. Andrews, "The Body as Property: Some Philosophical Reflections—A Response to J. F. Childress," *Transplantation Proceedings* 24, no. 5 (1992): 2150.

33. See the discussions in chapters 3 and 4 on safeguarding compensated donors and in chapter 1 on health risks to donors.

34. Michael J. Sandel, "Markets, Morals, and Civil Life," *Bulletin of the American Academy*, Summer 2005, 7, http://www.amacad.org/publications/bulletin/Summer2005/MarketsMoralsCivitLife.pdf (accessed December 26, 2007).

35. Kieran Healy, *Last Best Gifts: Altruism and the Market for Human Blood and Organs* (Chicago: University of Chicago Press, 2006), 92.

36. National Kidney Foundation, "Financial Incentives" (Consensus Conference, Controversies in Organ Donation, February 25–26, 1991), as cited in James F. Childress, "The Body as Property: Some Philosophical Reflections," *Transplantation Proceedings* 24, no. 5 (October 1992): 2146.

37. Arnold et al., "Financial Incentives for Cadaver Organ Donation," 1361.

38. Thomas A. Shannon, "The Kindness of Strangers: Organ Transplantation in a Capitalist Age," *Kennedy Institute of Ethics Journal* 11, no. 3 (September 2001): 302.

39. Childress, "The Body as Property," 2148.

40. T. Ashkenazi to Gabriel Danovitch, personal communication, May 7, 2006, cited in Gabriel M. Danovitch and Alan B. Leichtman, "Kidney Vending: The 'Trojan Horse' of Organ Transplantation," *Clinical Journal of the American Society of Nephrology* 1 (October 2006): 1133–35.

41. James Stacey Taylor, *Stakes and Kidneys: Why Markets in Human Body Parts are Morally Imperative* (Burlington, Vt.: Ashgate Publishing, 1988). For more on transplant tourism, see chapter 3.

42. Laura A. Siminoff and Kata Chillag, "The Fallacy of the 'Gift of Life,'" *Hastings Center Report* 29, no. 6 (November–December 1999): 34–41; Mary A. Dew, Galen E. Switzer, Andrea F. DiMartini, Larissa Myaskovsky, and Megan Crowley-Makota, "Psychosocial Aspects of Living Organ Donation," in *Living Donor Transplantation*, ed. Henkie P. Tan, Amadeo Marcos, and Ron Shapiro, 7–26 (New York: Informa Healthcare USA, 2007).

43. Roberta G. Simmons, Susan Klein Marine, Richard L. Simmons, *Gift of Life: The Effect of Organ Transplantation on Individual, Family, and Societal Dynamics*, 2d ed. (New York: Transaction Publishers, 1987).

44. Raphael J. Leo, Beth A. Smith, and DeAnna L. Mori, "Guidelines for Conducting a Psychiatric Evaluation of the Unrelated Kidney Donor," *Psychosomatics* 44, no. 6 (December 2003): 452–60.

45. Renee C. Fox and Judith P. Swazey, *Spare Parts: Organ Replacement in American Society* (New York: Oxford University Press, 1992).

46. Ibid., 40.

47. Cohen, "Public Policy and the Sale of Human Organs," 53.

48. Thomas E. Starzl, *The Puzzle People—Memoirs of a Transplant Surgeon* (Pittsburgh: University of Pittsburgh Press, 1992), 147.

49. Sheila M. Rothman and David J. Rothman, "The Hidden Cost of Organ Sale," *American Journal of Transplantation* 6 (2006): 1524–28. See chapter 7.

50. Danovitch and Leichtman, "Kidney Vending: The 'Trojan Horse' of Organ Transplantation."

51. A. Etzioni, "Organ Donation: A Communitarian Approach," *Kennedy Institute Journal of Ethics* 13, no. 1 (March 2003): 1.

52. Rothman and Rothman, "The Hidden Cost of Organ Sale."

53. Childress, "The Body as Property," 2146.

54. Charles Fruit, letter to the editor, *Wall Street Journal*, May 23, 2006.

55. Dorothy Hayes, letter to the editor, *New York Times*, May 19, 2006.

56. Michael Bourne, "The Power of the Selfless Gift," *Baltimore Sun*, September 21, 2006.

57. Virginia Postrel, "The National Kidney Foundation's Bad Math and Guilty Conscience," *Dynamist Blog*, http://www.dynamist.com/weblog/archives/002182.html (accessed December 24, 2007).

58. Dolph Chianchiano, personal communication with the author, March 10, 2008.

59. J. Andreoni, "Impure Altruism and Donations to Public Goods: A Theory of Warm-Glow Giving?" *Economic Journal* 100, no. 401 (June 1990): 464–77.

60. Paul Seabright, "Blood, Bribes and the Crowding-Out of Altruism by Financial Incentives," unpublished manuscript on file with IDEI, Université de Toulouse, February 8, 2002, http://idei.fr/doc/by/seabright/blood_bribes.pdf (accessed June 10, 2008).

61. See appendix C.

62. Healy, *Last Best Gifts*.

63. Charles Fruit, letter to the editor, *New York Times*, May 19, 2006.

64. Mark J. Cherry, *Kidney for Sale by Owner: Human Organs, Transplantation, and the Market* (Washington, D.C.: Georgetown University Press, 2005), 7.

Chapter 6: Altruism and Valuable Consideration in Organ Transplantation

1. National Organ Transplant Act (NOTA), Pub. L. No. 98–507, sec. 301 (1984): "It shall be unlawful for any person to knowingly acquire, receive, or otherwise transfer any human organ for valuable consideration for use in human transplantation if the transfer affects interstate commerce." See appendix A and chapter 8 for further information and discussion.

2. Transplantation Society, "Policy and Ethics," http://www.transplantation-soc.org/policy.php (accessed December 20, 2007).

3. Sheila M. Rothman and David J. Rothman, "The Hidden Cost of Organ Sale," *American Journal of Transplantation* 6 (2006): 1524.

4. Ibid.

5. See, for example, Lloyd Cohen, "Increasing the Supply of Transplant Organs: The Virtues of a Futures Market," *George Washington Law Review* 58 (1989): 1–51; Henry Hansmann, "The Economics and Ethics of Markets for Human Organs," *Journal of Health Policy, Politics and Law* 14 (1989): 57–85.

6. Institute of Medicine, *Organ Donation: Opportunities for Action* (Washington, D.C.: National Academies Press, 2006).

7. Ibid.

8. Vivekanand Jha and Kirpal S. Chugh, "The Case Against a Regulated System of Living Kidney Sales," *Nature Clinical Practice Nephrology* 2 (2006): 467.

9. Richard Titmuss, *The Gift Relationship: From Human Blood to Social Policy* (New York: Pantheon Books, 1971). Titmuss argued that "the commercialization of blood represses the expression of altruism [and] erodes the sense of community" (245).

10. I received this e-mail from Dr. Nirav Shah, then both a law and medical student at the University of Chicago, who was working in December 2006 in India: "The progress has a sinister side: a few months ago, a pernicious organ selling ring was cracked and revealed stories that would be harrowing even if fictional—scores of 'untouchables' goaded into selling kidneys for the benefit of wealthy foreigners tired of waiting lists at home. But in this case, the informed consent process yielded neither information nor consent. Sure, the organs were sold to foreigners but, in most cases, the 'sellers' got nothing in return for their kidneys other than a scar and a promise that payment would arrive once the doctors could confirm the organ wouldn't be rejected. Not surprisingly, all the donors were told that their organs had been rejected and that they wouldn't be paid."

11. Walter Graham (executive director of UNOS) to Francis L. Delmonico (president of UNOS), April 6, 2006 (hard copy on file with editor, S. Satel). Also see chapter 5.

12. Adam Smith, *The Wealth of Nations* (New York: Modern Library Edition, 1937), at 15.

13. For a vivid account of the risks of liver transplantation, see Laura Meckler, "The High Price of Keeping Dad Alive," *Wall Street Journal*, January 22, 2007, A1.

14. Henry Hansmann, "The Role of Nonprofit Enterprise," *Yale Law Journal* 89 (1980): 835; Edward L. Glaeser and Andrei Shleifer, "Not-for-Profit Entrepreneurs," *Journal of Public Economics* 81 (2001): 99. For exhaustive documentation of the frequent rescue attempts, too many of which go awry, see David Hyman, "Rescue Without Law: An Empirical Perspective on the Duty to Rescue," *Texas Law Review* 84 (2005): 653.

15. Organ Procurement and Transplantation Network, "Data: View Data Reports," http://www.optn.org/latestData/advancedData.asp (accessed January 4, 2008).

16. Alvin E. Roth, "Repugnance as a Constraint on Markets," *Journal of Economic Perspectives* 21, no. 3 (Summer 2007): 37.

17. Ibid., 46.

18. Robert S. Gaston, Gabriel M. Danovitch, Richard A. Epstein, Jeffrey P. Kahn, Arthur J. Matas, and Mark A. Schnitzler, "Limiting Financial Disincentives in Live Organ Donation: A Rational Solution to the Kidney Shortage," *American Journal of Transplantation* 6 (2006): 2548.

19. Mark D. Fox, "The Price is Wrong: The Moral Cost of Living Donor Inducements," *American Journal of Transplantation* 6, no. 11 (2006): 2529–30.

20. See LifeSharers, "LifeSharers: Organs for Organ Donors," http://www.lifesharers.org (accessed May 14, 2008). In the interest of full disclosure, I must mention that I am on the LifeSharers board and have signed up in the program.

21. For a variation on LifeSharers that also meets the NOTA requirements, see Mark S. Nadel and Carolina A. Nadel, "Using Reciprocity to Motivate Organ Donations," *Yale Journal of Health Policy, Law, and Ethics* 5 (2005): 293, 312–23, which seeks to give additional points within the UNOS framework to those who promise to donate organs. Once again, the proposal raises the prospect that parties who are most likely to commit are those who are likely to be organ recipients, so that the market remains perpetually out of equilibrium.

22. Mark D. Fox, Margaret R. Allee, and Gloria T. Taylor, "Opting for Equity," *American Journal of Bioethics* 4, no. 4 (2004): 15.

23. Sheldon Zink, Stacey Wertlieb, John Catalano, and Victor Marwin, "Examining the Potential Exploitation of UNOS Policies," *American Journal of Bioethics* 5 (2005): 8–9. The UNOS list sets the order in which individuals with end-stage renal disease are entitled to receive kidneys as the organs become available. This order depends in part on geography, in part on the time that a person gets on the list, and in part on other characteristics, such as compatibility and general fitness to receive an organ. Some sense of the complexity of these criteria is found on the UNOS website, which summarizes its waiting list policy as follows: "The Patient Waiting List contains information used by the computer system to match potential organ recipients with available organ donors. Waiting list data can be entered online into the waiting list database by the UNOS Organ Center staff or by registered UNOS transplant professional members. Renal candidate data elements

include name, gender, race, age, ABO blood group, number of previous transplants, peak and current panel reactive antibody (PRA) levels, acceptable donor characteristics, and patient human leukocyte antigens (HLAs). Information regarding non-renal candidates includes patient status codes (reflecting degree of medical urgency) for heart and liver, ABO blood group, patient age, gender, number of previous transplants, and acceptable donor characteristics. Each time a new patient is added to the waiting list, a Transplant Candidate Registration Form is generated for the member. When completed, this form adds additional clinical data about the potential transplant recipient." United Network for Organ Sharing, "Data: Data Collection," http://www.unos.org/data/about/collection.asp (accessed May 14, 2008).

24. For UNOS's ambivalent attitude, see Francis L. Delmonico (UNOS president) and Walter Graham (UNOS executive director), "Memorandum Addresses Federal Register to Solicit Comments on OPTN Oversight of Living Donor Guidelines," Organ Procurement and Transplantation Network news, January 23, 2006, www.optn.org/news/ newsDetail.asp?id=526 (accessed March 27, 2008).

25. Arthur L. Caplan, Sheldon Zink, and Stacey L. Wertlieb, "Jumping to the Front of the Line for an Organ Transplant Is Unfair," *Chicago Tribune*, September 1, 2004; Zink et al., "Examining the Potential Exploitation of UNOS Policies," 6–10.

26. Christopher Snowbeck, "Publicity Campaigns Seeking Organ Donations Raise Ethics Questions," *Pittsburgh Post-Gazette*, August 23, 2004, http://www.postgazette.com/pg/04236/366176.stm (accessed March 27, 2008).

27. Rob Stein, "Search for Transplant Organs Becomes a Web Free-for-All," *Washington Post*, September 23, 2005, A01.

28. Lainie Ross et al., "Ethics of a Paired-Kidney Exchange Program," *New England Journal of Medicine* 336 (1997): 1752.

29. Francis L. Delmonico, "Reply to Letter to the Editor," *New England Journal of Medicine* 351 (2004): 937.

30. Arthur J. Matas, "Policy Analysis—A Regulated System of Compensation for Living Kidney Donation: Rationale and Concern" (Washington, D.C.: Cato Institute, 2007). See also Matas, "Why We Should Develop a Regulated System of Kidney Sales," *Clinical Journal of the American Society of Nephrology* 1 (2006): 1129.

31. Ibid.

32. Arthur J. Matas, "A Gift of Life Deserves Compensation: How to Increase Living Kidney Donation with Realistic Incentives," CATO Policy Analysis, no. 64, November 7, 2007: 5, http://www.cato.org/pubs/pas/pa-604.pdf.

33. *Jackson v. Seymour*, 71 S.E.2d 181 (Va. 1952).

34. See chapter 2.

35. Arthur J. Matas and Mark A. Schnitzler, "Payment for Living Donor (Vendor) Kidneys: A Cost-Effectiveness Analysis," *American Journal of Transplantation* 4 (2004): 216.

36. For one stark account, see Benjamin Hippen, "The Case for Kidney Markets," *New Atlantis* 14 (2006): 47–61, http://www.thenewatlantis.com/archive/14/hippen.htm (accessed March 27, 2008).

37. This estimate is given that almost half of the dialysis population is over sixty-five years old, and that the majority of those will die within five years of starting dialysis. See U.S. Renal Data System, *2006 Annual Data Report Reference* Tables, 112, table D.11; 298, table 1.4; 300, table 1.6; and 301, table 1.7, http://www.usrds.org/reference.htm (accessed May 14, 2008).

38. Jason Riis et al., "Ignorance of Hedonic Adaptation to Hemodialysis: A Study Using Ecological Momentary Assessment," *Journal of Experimental Psychology* 134 (2005): 3.

39. Renee D. Goodwin, Andrej Marusic, and Christina W. Hoven, "Suicide Attempts in the United States: The Role of Physical Illness," *Social Science & Medicine* 56 (2003): 1783–88.

40. Lionel U. Mailloux et al., "Death by Withdrawal from Dialysis: A 20-Year Clinical Experience," *Journal of the American Society of Nephrology* 3 (1993): 1631; Lewis M. Cohen et al., "Practical Considerations in Dialysis Withdrawal," *Journal of the American Medical Association* 289 (2003): 2113; Michael J. McCarthy, "The Choice: Years on Dialysis Brought Joe Mole to a Cross Roads," *Wall Street Journal*, November 3, 2005; Friedrich K. Port et al., "Discontinuation of Dialysis Therapy as a Cause of Death," *American Journal of Nephrology* 9 (1989): 145–49; Silja Neu and Carl M. Kjellstrand, "Stopping Long-Term Dialysis. An Empirical Study of Withdrawal of Life-Supporting Treatment," *New England Journal of Medicine* 314 (1986): 14–20; John E. Leggat Jr. et al., "An Analysis of Risk Factors for Withdrawal from Dialysis before Death," *Journal of the American Society of Nephrology* 8 (1997): 1755–63; K. Bajwa, E. Szabo, and C. M. Kjellstrand, "A Prospective Study of Risk Factors and Decision-Making in Discontinuation of Dialysis," *Archives of Internal Medicine* 156 (1991): 2571–77; Alan S. Kliger and Fredric O. Finkelstein, "Which Patients Choose to Stop Dialysis?" *Nephrology Dialysis Transplantation* 18 (2003): 869–71.

41. Leggat et al., "An Analysis of Risk Factors"; Mailloux et al., "Death by Withdrawal from Dialysis"; Cohen et al., "Practical Considerations in Dialysis Withdrawal." Needless to say, these figures are difficult to interpret. Persons on dialysis suffer from painful or debilitating conditions, such as advanced diabetes, which might prompt withdrawal from treatment even by those who can tolerate dialysis. McCarthy, "The Choice."

42. In 2005 there were eighty thousand to ninety thousand deaths on dialysis. Five thousand to seven thousand of the deaths were deemed voluntary withdrawal, but only seventy to eighty were labeled as suicides. Paul W. Eggers (program director for kidney and urology epidemiology, National Institute of Diabetes and Digestive and Kidney Diseases), e-mail communication to the author, July 24, 2008.

43. Manjula Kurella et al., "Suicide in the United States End-Stage Renal Disease Program," *Journal of the American Society of Nephrology* 16 (2005): 774–81. "The risk of death from suicide in ESRD patients is greater than that in the general population," the authors write. "However, it is not nearly as high as was suggested by earlier data that lumped death by withdrawal from dialysis together with death from suicide."

44. Harry S. Abram, Gordon L. Moore, and Frederic B. Westervelt Jr., "Suicidal Behavior in Chronic Dialysis Patients," *American Journal of Psychiatry* 127 (1971): 1199–1204.

45. Neu and Kjellstrand, "Stopping Long-Term Dialysis."

46. Kevin Murphy and Robert Topel, "The Cost of Living: How Much Would You Pay to Live a Longer and Healthier Life?" *Chicago GSB*, Chicago Graduate School of Business, Spring 2000, http://www.chicagogsb.edu/magazine/S00/research1.html (accessed March 27, 2008).

47. Gabriel C. Oniscu et al., "How Great is the Survival Advantage of Transplantation Over Dialysis in Elderly Patients?" *Nephrology Dialysis Transplantation* 19 (2004): 945. In patients more than sixty years old, the authors found a significantly lower risk of death and a longer life expectancy after listing with a transplant. People with transplants lived an average 8.17 years versus 4.32 years for those on dialysis.

48. See chapter 2.

49. U.S. Renal Data System, *2007 Annual Data Report*, 162, www.usrds.org/2006/pdf/07_tx_06.pdf (accessed May 14, 2008).

50. "Renal Transplant Patients Have a Good Quality of Life," *Drug & Therapy Perspectives* 11, no. 8 (1998): 14.

51. Matas and Schnitzler, "Payment for Living Donor (Vendor) Kidneys," 216, 219. The authors, a transplant surgeon and an economist, found the total cost of care during the first year after a living-donor transplant to be $72,693 and the annual cost thereafter to be $12,814.

52. Ibid., 218, table 1.

53. For some evidence of the grueling family pressures of liver transplantation, see Meckler, "The High Price of Keeping Dad Alive," A1.

54. William H. Bay and Lee A. Hebert, "The Living Donor in Kidney Transplantation," *Annals of Internal Medicine* 106 (1987): 719; Arthur J. Matas, Stephen T. Bartlett, Alan B. Leichtman, and Francis L. Delmonico, "Morbidity and Mortality after Living Kidney Donation, 1999–2001: Survey of United States Transplant Centers," *American Journal of Transplantation* 3 (2003): 830. The morbidity figure falls below 2 percent. See also chapter 1, above.

55. Robert Gaston, communication with the author, January 8, 2007.

56. Sheila M. Rothman and David J. Rothman, "The Hidden Cost of Organ Sale," *American Journal of Transplantation* 6 (2006): 1528.

57. Gabriel M. Danovitch and Alan B. Leichtman, "Kidney Vending: The 'Trojan Horse' of Organ Transplantation," *Clinical Journal of the American Society of Nephrology* 1 (2006): 1133–35.

58. See also chapter 7.

59. See chapter 5.

60. Kieran Healy, *Last Best Gifts: Altruism and the Market for Human Blood and Organs* (Chicago: University of Chicago Press, 2006), 92.

61. Jeremy Shearmur, "In Defense of Commercial Provision of Blood: Reactions to Voluntarism in the United States National Blood Policy in the Early 1970s," *Journal of Value Inquiry* 40, nos. 2–3 (2006): 279–95.

62. Giving blood for plasma takes about two hours, while giving whole blood takes under one hour. According to the U.S. Government Accountability Office (GAO), the

payment is required as an incentive for donors to sit at the collection site for at least double the time it takes to make a whole-blood donation. U.S. Government Accountability Office, *Blood Supply: FDA Oversight and Remaining Issues of Safety*, GAO/PEMD-97-1 (Washington, D.C.: U.S. Government Printing Office, 1997), 26, quoted in Joel Schwartz, "Blood and Altruism—Richard M. Titmuss' Criticism of the Commercialization of Blood," *Public Interest* 136 (Summer 1999): 46.

Chapter 7: Crowding Out, Crowding In, and Financial Incentives for Organ Procurement

1. The origin of the term "crowding out" is not entirely clear, and perhaps less relevant than the fact that the phenomenon has been a topic of discussion in the economics literature dating back to Adam Smith's *The Wealth of Nations*. For a broad overview of the history of the term, see Roger W. Spencer and William P. Yohe, "The 'Crowding Out' of Private Expenditures by Fiscal Policy Actions," *Review* (Federal Reserve Bank of St. Louis), October 1970, 12–24. Spencer and Yohe identify the term in a textbook of macroeconomics published in 1968.

2. Richard Titmuss, *The Gift Relationship: From Human Blood to Social Policy* (London: Allen & Unwin, 1971); Jeffrey M. Prottas, "Buying Human Organs—Evidence that Money Doesn't Change Everything," *Transplantation* 53, no. 6 (June 1992): 1371–73; Sheila M. Rothman and David J. Rothman, "The Hidden Cost of Organ Sale," *American Journal of Transplantation* 6, no. 7 (July 2006): 1524–28. It should be noted that the term "crowding out," as a matter of displacing altruism (without necessarily reducing the total supply of blood), does not appear in *The Gift Relationship*, though the book discusses the phenomenon itself at length.

3. "Only about 7 percent of all donations in the United States are derived from voluntary donors who regard their donation as a free gift to strangers," Titmuss, *Gift Relationship*, 111.

4. Ibid., 88–89.

5. Ibid., 34–35.

6. Ibid., 56.

7. Harvey M. Sapolsky and Stan N. Finkelstein, "Blood Policy Revisited—A New Look at 'The Gift Relationship,'" *Public Interest* 46 (Winter 1977): 17.

8. Douglas Starr, *Blood: An Epic History of Medicine and Commerce* (New York: Alfred A. Knopf, 1998). It appears, for example, that Titmuss significantly overestimated the segment of the American blood supply system that was commercial and overstated the amount of collected blood that expired and thus went unused. See Alvin W. Drake, Stan N. Finkelstein, and Harvey M. Sapolsky, *The American Blood Supply: Issues and Policies of Blood Donation* (Cambridge, Mass.: MIT Press, 1982).

9. Titmuss, *Gift Relationship*, 94–95.

10. Ibid., 78–84. Cash payment of a premium was an alternative to donating for this purpose, a point heavily criticized by Titmuss.

11. Ibid., 111.

12. Ibid., 94, table 1.

13. Ibid., 130-31.

14. Ibid., 307.

15. Ibid., appendix 6, 307.

16. Ibid., appendix 6, 309–15.

17. Ibid., 238–39.

18. Factor VIII is a vital component of blood needed for clotting. It is required for the treatment of hemophilia A, a bleeding disorder.

19. Starr, *Blood*, 240. Blood fractionation is the process of separating whole blood into its component parts.

20. Figure from a précis of *The Blood Industry*, a business strategy report published in November 2005, http://www.piribo.com/publications/medical_devices/blood_industry.html (accessed June 26, 2008).

21. Titmuss, *Gift Relationship*, 223.

22. Ibid., 242.

23. Kenneth Arrow, "Gifts and Exchanges," *Philosophy and Public Affairs* 4 (Summer 1972): 351; see also Raymond Solow, "Blood and Thunder" (review of Titmuss's *The Gift Relationship*), *Yale Law Journal* 80, no. 8 (July 1971): 1704; and Nathan Glazer, "Blood," *Public Interest* 24 (Summer 1971): 89.

24. Arrow, "Gifts and Exchanges," 350

25. This insight is most thoroughly developed in Kieran Healy, *Last Best Gifts: Altruism and the Market for Human Blood and Organs* (Chicago: University of Chicago Press, 2006).

26. R. G. Strauss et al., "Concurrent Comparison of the Safety of Paid Cytopheresis and Volunteer Whole Blood Donors," *Transfusion* 34 (1994): 116–21; R. E. Domen, "Paid-versus-Volunteer Blood Donation in the United States: A Historical Review," *Transfusion Medicine Review* 9 (1995): 53–59; R. D. Aach and R. A. Kahn, "Post-Transfusion Hepatitis: Current Perspectives," *Annals of Internal Medicine* 92 (1980): 539–46.

27. Sapolsky and Finkelstein, "Blood Policy Revisited," 18.

28. Ross D. Eckert, "AIDS and the Blood Bankers," *Regulation* 10, no. 5 (September/October 1986): 15, 20.

29. Drake, *The American Blood Supply*, 38

30. Ibid., 40

31. R. G. Strauss, "Blood Donations, Safety and Incentives," *Transfusion* 41, no. 2 (2001): 165–67.

32. Healy, *Last Best Gifts*.

33. M. Simons, "Courtroom Anguish as France Tries 4 over Tainted Blood," *New York Times*, July 31, 1992.

34. Starr, *Blood*, 355.

35. Douglas Clibourn (chief executive officer, Zymequest, Beverly, Mass.), personal communication with the authors, December 5, 2007.

36. Plasma donors are paid because giving blood for plasma takes twice as long as giving whole blood; see chapter 6.

37. U.S. House of Representatives, Committee on Energy and Commerce, Subcommittee on Oversight and Investigations, *Assessing Initiatives to Increase Organ Donations: Hearing Before the Subcommittee on Oversight and Investigations of the House Committee on Energy and Commerce*, 108th Cong., 1st sess., June 3, 2003, statement of Francis L. Delmonico, MD, for the National Kidney Foundation, 66.

38. Rothman and Rothman, "Hidden Cost of Organ Sale"; Uri Gneezy and Aldo Rustichini, "A Fine Is a Price," *Journal of Legal Studies* 29, no. 1 (2000): 1–17.

39. Rothman and Rothman, "Hidden Cost of Organ Sale."

40. U. Gneezy and A. Rustichini, "Pay Enough or Don't Pay at All," *Quarterly Journal of Economics* 115, no. 2 (2000): 791–810.

41. U. Gneezy, Werner Guth, and Frank Verboven, "Presents or Investments? An Experimental Analysis," *Journal of Economic Psychology* 21, no. 5 (2000): 491.

42. Gneezy and Rustichini, "Pay Enough or Don't Pay at All."

43. Carl Mellström and Magnus Johannesson, "Crowding Out in Blood Donation: Was Titmuss Right?" Paper No. 180, Department of Economics, Göteborg University, 2006, http://www.handels.gu.se/epc/archive/00004448/01/gunwpe0180.pdf (accessed June 26, 2008); Gneezy and Rustichini, "Pay Enough or Don't Pay at All"; Paul Seabright, "Blood, Bribes and the Crowding-Out of Altruism by Financial Incentives," unpublished manuscript on file with IDEI Toulouse, February 8, 2002, http://idei.fr/doc/by/seabright/blood_bribes.pdf (accessed June 26, 2008); Healy, *Last Best Gifts*; Bruno S. Frey and Lorenz Goette, "Does Pay Motivate Volunteers?" Working Paper iewwp007, Institute for Empirical Research in Economics, University of Zurich, June 11, 1999, http://ideas.repec.org/p/zur/iewwpx/007.html (accessed July 2, 2008). The authors administered a survey to volunteers and found that those offered payment worked fewer hours than those not compensated. B. S. Frey and F. Oberholzer-Gee, "The Cost of Price Incentives: An Empirical Analysis of Motivation Crowding-Out," *American Economic Review* 87, no. 4 (1997): 746–55. The research team surveyed Swiss residents to gauge their willingness to accept a repository of nuclear waste in their neighborhood. They noted that willingness dropped by one-third to one-half when compensation was offered; increasing proposed compensation by several thousand dollars could not reverse the effect.

44. Dan Ariely, Anat Bracha, and Stephan Meier, "Doing Good or Doing Well? Image Motivation and Monetary Incentives in Behaving Prosocially," Working Papers 07-9, Federal Reserve Bank of Boston, 2007, http://ideas.repec.org/s/fip/fedbwp.html (accessed May 25, 2008).

45. Healy, *Last Best Gifts*.

46. Seabright, "Blood, Bribes and the Crowding-Out of Altruism"; Healy, *Last Best Gifts*; Mellström and Johannesson, "Crowding Out in Blood Donation."

47. Gneezy and Rustichini, "Pay Enough or Don't Pay at All," 119.

48. Gabriel Danovitch, "Cultural Barriers to Kidney Transplantation: A New Frontier," *Transplantation* 84, no. 4 (2007): 462–63.

49. Benjamin E. Hippen, "A Modest Approach to a New Frontier: Commentary on Danovitch," *Transplantation* 84, no. 4 (2007): 464–66.

50. Benjamin E. Hippen, "Organ Sales and Moral Travails: Lessons from the Living Kidney Vendor Program in Iran," *Cato Policy Analysis* No. 614, Cato Institute, March 20, 2008, http://www.cato.org/pub_display.php?pub_id=9273 (accessed July 2, 2008).

51. One line of evidence supporting the prediction that compensation will increase the supply of kidneys comes from medical schools. Students required to perform dissections in anatomy class must work with intact cadavers. Because the law does not prohibit medical schools from compensating families who allow their loved ones' bodies to be used for this purpose, the schools can do so by covering the cost of cremation or burial. Plausibly, this is why the United States has a surplus of cadavers. The assumption is bolstered by the observation of economists David Harrington and Edward Sayre that, all else being equal, states in which cremation is more expensive have higher rates of whole-cadaver donation (presumably because families can save more money). Ideally, we would want to know if there was a time when families donated loved ones' bodies just as they do with organs today. That would permit a specific conclusion about crowding out. While this is not a comparison we have the data to make, the price sensitivity observed by Harrington and Sayre implies that families respond more enthusiastically when the amount of the incentives offered is greater. David E. Harrington and Edward A. Sayre, "Paying for Bodies, But Not for Organs," *Regulation* 29, no. 4 (Winter 2006–7): 14–19.

52. U. Gneezy and J. List, "Putting Behavioral Economics to Work: Testing for Gift Exchange in Labor Markets Using Field Experiments," *Econometrica* 74, no. 5 (2006): 1365–84, especially 1366–67.

53. G. M. Danovitch, "Cultural Barriers," and B. E. Hippen, "A Modest Approach."

54. W. Harmon and F. Delmonico, "Payment for Kidneys: A Government-Regulated System Is Not Ethically Achievable," *Clinical Journal of the American Society of Nephrology* 1, no. 6 (November 2006): 1146–47.

55. The very low rate of organ procurement from deceased donors in Australia as compared to European countries has been attributed in part to the scarcity of intensive care resources there. See Laura Tiernan, "Australia: $50,000 for a Kidney? Doctor's Proposal Highlights Desperate Health, Social Crisis," World Socialist Web Site, May 16, 2008, http://www.wsws.org/articles/2008/may2008/kidn- m16.shtml.

56. See, for example, BBC2, "Iran Kidney Sale," *This World*, October 31, 2006, http://news. bbc.co.uk/2/hi/programmes/this_world/6080328.stm (accessed January 4, 2008).

57. Benjamin Hippen, "Organ Sales and Moral Travails."

58. Harmon and Delmonico, "Payment for Kidneys."

59. Hippen, "Organ Sales and Moral Travails."

60. Ibid.

61. Healy, *Last Best Gifts*, 42.

Chapter 8: Rethinking Federal Organ Transplantation Policy: Model Legislation for State Waivers

1. See 42 U.S.C. secs. 273–74 (2006); the Organ Procurement Transplantation Network was established out of 42 U.S.C. sec. 274 (a)–(b) (2006). See also appendix A.

2. University of Michigan Law Faculty, "Memorial Resolution by the University of Michigan Law Faculty Concerning E. Blythe Stason," *Michigan Law Review* 71, no. 3 (January 1973): 451–58. Stason also served as the Frank C. Rand Distinguished Professor of Law at Vanderbilt University during the drafting of the UAGA.

3. Ibid.

4. E. B. Stason, "The Uniform Anatomical Gift Act," *Business Law* 23 (1968): 927.

5. See act of June 12, 1967, ch. 353, 1967 Mass. Acts 202, 202 (repealed 1971), prohibiting the sale of organs, body parts, and tissues after death. See also law of August 1, 1968, ch. 429, sec. 7, 56 Del. Laws, 1773, 1773 (1967; repealed 1970); law of May 20, 1967, ch. 94, sec. 1, 1967 Hawaii laws 91, 91 (repealed 1969), prohibiting the sale of bodies after death; law of April 24, 1961, ch. 315, sec. 1, 11961 Md. Laws 397, 398 (repealed 1968); law of April 22, 1964, ch. 702, sec. 1, 1964 N.Y. Laws 1827, 1828 (repealed 1971). Statutes cited in Susan Hankin Denise, "Note, Regulating the Sale of Human Organs," *Virginia Law Review* 71, no. 6 (September 1985): 1022–23.

6. See, for example, Stason, "Uniform Anatomical Gift Act," 921–24.

7. Ibid.

8. Denise, "Regulating the Sale of Human Organs," 1015; Nicholas Wade, "The Crisis in Human Spare Parts," *New York Times*, October 4, 1983, A26.

9. Lloyd Cohen, "Increasing the Supply of Transplant Organs: The Virtues of a Futures Market," *George Washington Law Review* 58, no. 1 (November 1989): 7.

10. Keith Mueller, "The National Transplant Act of 1984: Congressional Response to Changing Biotechnology," *Policy Studies Review* 8, no. 2 (Winter 1988): 346, 350.

11. Ibid.

12. Section 301 of NOTA.

13. A superficial reading of section 301 would seem to suggest that by banning valuable consideration only for transactions that affect interstate commerce, Congress left room for states to experiment with compensation programs that did not involve the crossing of state lines by organ donors or recipients. Landmark Supreme Court cases in the twentieth century, however, expanded the definition of interstate commerce to include anything whatsoever that is traded across state lines to or from a business or other institution. For all intents and purposes, all commerce is now deemed interstate, including that in which a transplant program would have to engage to acquire drugs, surgical instruments, diagnostic equipment, food for patients, bed linens, office supplies, cleaning agents, and so forth, and so the federal ban on valuable consideration applies to all such programs.

14. Virginia was the first state to ban the sale of organs from living or dead donors. See Va. Code, sec. 32.1–289.1 (1985).

15. University of Michigan Law Faculty, "Memorial Resolution."

16. Pennsylvania State Legislature, Probate, Estates, & Fiduciaries Code (20 PA.C.S.) Amend Act of 1994, P.L. 655, no. 102.

17. Cindy Bryce, Laura Siminoff, Peter Ubel, Howard Nathan, Arthur Caplan, and Robert Arnold, "Do Incentives Matter? Providing Benefits to Families of Organ Donors," *American Journal of Transplantation* 5, no. 12 (December 2005): 2999–3008.

18. Christopher Snowbeck, "Committee Plan to Reward Families for Relatives' Organ Donations," *Pittsburgh Post-Gazette*, June 10, 1999, B7.

19. Sheryl G. Stolberg, "Pennsylvania Set to Break Taboo on Reward for Organ Donations," *New York Times*, May 6, 1999, A1.

20. A committee of fifteen was appointed by the governor to evaluate the ethical, moral, and legal issues associated with the act. Pennsylvania State Department of Health, Act 102 of 1994, July 20, 2006, http://www.dsf.health.state.pa.us/health/cwp/view.asp?A=174&Q=244786 (accessed November 13, 2007).

21. Howard Nathan (president and chief executive officer, Gift of Life Donor Program, Philadelphia), personal conversation with the author, October 24, 2007.

22. Memo dated January 5, 2001 from Jon L. Nelson, director, Health Research and Services Administration, to the Honorable Joseph A. Petarca, House of Representatives, Commonwealth of Pennsylvania (on file with author); Christopher Snowbeck, "Organ Donor Funeral Aid Scrapped," *Pittsburgh Post-Gazette*, February 1, 2002.

23. Ethics Committee of the American Society of Transplant Surgeons, "Financial Incentives for Cadaver Organ Donation: An Ethical Reappraisal," *Transplantation* 73, no. 8 (April 2002): 1361–67.

24. See the No Child Left Behind Act and Title IV-A of the Social Security Act.

25. See U.S. Department of Health and Human Services, Office of the Assistant Secretary for Planning and Evaluation, "State Welfare Waivers: An Overview," aspe.hhs.gov/HSP/isp/waiver2/waivers.htm (accessed September 17, 2007).

26. Ibid.

27. Tommy Thompson (governor of Wisconsin, 1987–2001), "The Good News about Welfare Reform: Wisconsin's Success Story," speech to the Heritage Foundation, March 6, 1997, http://www.heritage.org/Research/Welfare/HL593.cfm (accessed January 17, 2008)

28. U.S. Department of Health and Human Services, "Five States Awarded New Child Welfare Waivers," June 2006, http://cbexpress.acf.hhs.gov/articles.cfm?issue_id=2006-06&article_id=1166 (accessed September 1, 2007).

29. Ibid.

30. Ibid.

31. Cody's Law (Assembly Bill 477) was named after Cody Monroe, an eight-year-old from Menasha, Wisconsin, whose life was saved by a kidney transplant from his father. Marty Monroe, a truck driver, had to miss twelve weeks of work following the surgery, costing the family about $6,000 in lost wages. Kawanza L. Griffin, "Donors Get Tax Break," *Milwaukee Journal Sentinel*, January 30, 2004. Cody's Law, which was enacted in

January 2004, was the first in the nation to offer a tax benefit to living donors. While the number of living donations in Wisconsin went up by over 20 percent in 2004–5, the nature of the data makes it difficult to determine how much of the increase was the direct result of the new law. Subsequent years saw the rate of living donations settle back to its pre-Cody level. Data from Michigan, one of eleven states that currently offer a $10,000 tax deduction, suggest that the tax benefit has actually made little difference in the number of transplants performed there—in contrast to Utah, which enjoyed an almost 30 percent increase in living donations after 2005, the first year of its tax credit law. Amy Olszewski (government liaison for Michigan Gift of Life), personal communication with the author and Sally Satel, November 13 and 27, 2007; Alex McDonald (director of public education/public relations, Intermountain Donor Services), telephone interview with the author, November 13, 2007.

32. Steven Wieckert (Wisconsin state representative), telephone interview with the author, November 14, 2007. Wieckert would like to try bolder moves to increase donations—perhaps conduct a pilot study in which kidney donors would receive substantial compensation, not merely reimbursement.

33. Among the states with tax incentive laws are Wisconsin, Utah, Mississippi, New York, Ohio, North Dakota, Oklahoma, and Idaho.

34. U.S. Department of Health and Human Services, Centers for Medicare and Medicaid Services, "Details for MMA Section 646 Physician Hospital Collaboration Demonstration," http://www.cms.hhs.gov/DemoProjectsEvalRpts/MD/itemdetail. asp?filterType=none&filterByDID=-99&sortByDID=3&sortOrder%20= ascending&itemID=CMS1186653 (accessed November 22, 2007).

35. See chapters 5, 6, and 7.

Conclusion

1. *DutchNews.nl*, "Thousands Sign Up as Organ Donors," June 4, 2007, http://www.dutchnews.nl/news/archives/2007/06/thousands_sign_up_as_organ_don. php (accessed March 18, 2008).

2. Dr. Gert van Dijk, author of one of the papers, said they were asked to write the report in the summer of 2007. Gert van Dijk, personal communication with the author, March 26, 2008.

3. Gert van Dijk and Medard T. Hilhorst, *Financial Incentives for Organ Donation: An Investigation of the Ethical Issues*, Centre for Ethics and Health, The Hague, 2007, http://www.ceg.nl/data/download/Orgaandonatie_huisstijl_eng_def.pdf (accessed June 5, 2008).

4. Nicola Smith and Aaron Gray-Block, "Dutch May Give Financial Reward to Kidney Donors," *London Times*, November 19, 2007.

5. Medard Hilhorst (professor, Department of Medical Ethics, Erasmus Medical Center), personal communication with the author, March 21, 2008. In May 2007, prior to the airing of *The Big Donor Show*, one of the largest firms of undertakers in the Netherlands announced it would offer families a modest reduction in the cost of

funerals if they agreed to bequeath their loved ones' organs. The plan followed a call from the Dutch Kidney Foundation, which was seeking new strategies to expand the organ donor pool in the light of the increasing unwillingness of living people to donate. Tony Sheldon, "Undertakers Offer Cash Incentive for Organ Donation in an Attempt to Encourage Donors," *British Medical Journal* 334, no. 7604 (June 2007): 1131. In December 2008, four major Dutch insurers agreed to discount annual fees for organ donors. "Dutch health care insurers to give discount to organ donors," *The Earth Times*, December 1, 2008, http://www.earthtimes.org/articles/show/244141,dutch-health-care-insurers-to-give-discount-to-organ-donors.html.

6. P. K. Abdul Ghafour, "Organ Donation Law to Help Thousands," *Arab News*, October 15, 2006, http://www.arabnews.com/?page=1&section=0&article=88218&d=15&m=10&y=2006 (accessed June 5, 2008).

7. *NewsTrack India*, "Organ Transplant to Be Legalised: Incentive and Other Benefits for the Donor," January 31, 2008, www.newstrackindia.com/newsdetails/2245 (accessed March 22, 2008).

8. Singapore Ministry of Health, "Organ Trading," press release, July 21, 2008, response to question no. 654 by Dr. Lam Pin Min, http://www.moh.gov.sg/mohcorp/parliamentaryqa.aspx?id=19598 (accessed July 23, 2008).

9. First, they must counter the misguided, if heartfelt, sentiments of individuals such as Luc Noel of the World Health Organization, who believes that "there are two prevailing concepts of transplantation. One relies on money and leads to increased inequality, besides putting a price on the integrity of the body and human dignity. The second is based on solidarity and the donor's sole motivation to save a life." Quoted by Paul Garwood, "Dilemma over Live-Donor Transplantation" *Bulletin of the World Health Organization* 85, no. 1 (January 2007), http://www.who.int/bulletin/volumes/85/1/07-020107/en/index.html (accessed June 5, 2008). In the debate over incentives, rhetoric touting false choices—genuine altruism versus rapacious black markets—is often accompanied by the raising of straw men. "Payments would exploit the most vulnerable members of our society, with the degree of exploitation influenced by gender, ethnicity, and the social status of the vendor. This exploitation has been the experience of a black market for organs throughout the world," a spokesman for the National Kidney Foundation told Congress. U.S. House of Representatives, Committee on Energy and Commerce, Subcommittee on Oversight and Investigation, *Assessing Initiatives to Increase Organ Donations*, 108th Cong., 1st sess., June 3, 2003, statement of Francis Delmonico, 51–54. Authors of an article invoking "the Trojan horse" of organ transplantation asserted, "We are confident that [the] proponents of a kidney vending system in the United States do not want to see the abuse of kidney sellers that is so common in the third world." Gabriel M. Danovitch and Alan B. Leichtman, "Kidney Vending: The 'Trojan Horse' of Organ Transplantation," *Clinical Journal of the American Society of Nephrology* 1, no. 6 (November 2006): 1133–35. While such exploitation and abuse do, in fact, take place in some parts of the world, they would be avoided in a well-regulated,

legal system of donor compensation, as authors of this book have demonstrated (see, especially, chapters 3 and 4). Indeed, the black markets themselves would disappear as safe and legitimate means for acquiring organs rendered them superfluous.

10. "Sale of organs is a zero-sum game in which any advantage of one participant necessarily leads to disadvantage to one or more of the others. The organ recipient is the only one who stands a chance for gain (organ brokers, surgeons, and hospitals notwithstanding)." David J. Rothman, "Ethical and Social Consequences of Selling a Kidney," *Journal of the American Medical Association* 288, no. 13 (October 2002): 1640–41.

11. Mark J. Piacentini, letter to the editor, *Medical Economics* 81, no. 17 (September 3, 2004), http://medicaleconomics.modernmedicine.com/memag/ModernMedicine+Now/Letters-to-the-Editors/ArticleStandard/Article/detail/120979 (accessed June 26, 2008).

12. Current UNOS policy allows anonymous donors to determine where, though not to whom, their kidneys go: "There may exist a presumption that [nondirected organs from living donors] may be applied for the exclusive benefit of the center's patients." OPTN/UNOS Ethics Committee, "Living Non-Directed Organ Donation," http://unos.org/resources/bioethics.asp?index=1 (accessed March 24, 2008).

13. National Kidney Foundation, "About the National Kidney Foundation," http://www.kidney.org/transplantation/livingDonors/index.cfm (accessed June 12, 2008).

14. John Davis (chief executive officer, National Kidney Foundation) to Christopher DeMuth (president, American Enterprise Institute), May 26, 2006, http://www.dynamist.com/weblog/aaa/NKF%20letter.pdf (accessed April 1, 2008).

15. See appendix A.

16. Charles Fruit, letter to the editor, *Wall Street Journal*, May 23, 2006. The sentiment was reiterated by Dolph Chianchiano, senior vice president for health policy and research at the NKF. He said that the NKF Family Donor Council (comprised of families who have donated loved ones' organs or their own) believes that compensating donors would "cheapen the gift." Personal communication with the author, March 10, 2008. This was discussed in chapter 5.

17. Thomas Peters, MD (member, AAKP Board of Directors), personal communication with the author, June 10, 2008.

18. Ibid., 84

19. U.S. House of Representatives, Committee on Energy and Commerce, Subcommittee on Oversight and Investigation, *Assessing Initiatives to Increase Organ Donations*. See 22–23 regarding the AOPO and 84 regarding UNOS.

20. American Medical Association, "Financial Incentives Could Improve Organ Donation and Reduce Donor-Recipient Gap," June 16, 2008, http://www.ama-assn.org/ama/pub/category/18674.html (accessed June 26, 2008).

21. U.S. House of Representatives, Committee on Energy and Commerce, Subcommittee on Health and the Environment, *Hearings on the National Organ Transplant Act*, 98th Cong., 1st sess., July 1983, statement of Representative Albert Gore

Jr., 9–10. The bill, H.R. 2856 (108th Cong., 1st sess., July 24, 2003), which was to authorize the secretary of health and human services to carry out demonstration projects to increase the supply of organs donated for human transplantation, had the support of no Republicans and five Democrats. Cosponsors were representatives Donna M. Christensen (D-VI), Martin Frost (D-TX), Rush D. Holt, (D-NJ), Donald M. Payne (D-NJ), and Vic Snyder (D-AR).

22. See appendix A for descriptions of bills and draft bills introduced since 1999 by Representatives Hansen, Smith, Greenwood, and Norwood, and Senator Frist.

23. Draft of bill on file with author; intent of bill articulated in bill summary drafted by Senator Specter's staff, on file with author.

24. E. Williams, B. Reyes-Akinbileje, K. Swendiman, *Congressional Research Service Report for Congress: Living Organ Donation and Valuable Consideration*, Washington, D.C.: Congressional Research Service, March 8, 2007; Office of Legal Counsel, U.S. Department of Justice, "Legality of Alternative Organ Donation Practices under 42 U.S.C § 274e," March 28, 2007, http://www.usdoj.gov/olc/2007/organtransplant.pdf.

25. Letter from AAKP, Roberta Wager, President, dated Sept. 22, 2008 (on file with author); Letter from AST, Barbara Murphy MD, President, dated Sept. 22, 2008 (on file with author).

Appendix A

1. Sullivan Group, "The Uniform Anatomical Gift Act of 1968," http://www.thesullivangroup.com/physician_law_review/anatomical_gifts/anatomical_2_historical.html (accessed October 4, 2007).

2. Uniform Law Commission, National Conference of Commissioners on Uniform State Laws, "New Revision to the Rules Governing Organ Donations Approved," press release, July 13, 2006, http://www.nccusl.org/Update/DesktopModules/NewsDisplay.aspx?ItemID=164 (accessed October 4, 2007).

3. Robyn S. Shapiro, "Legal Issues in Payment of Living Donors for Solid Organs," *Human Rights*, American Bar Association, Spring 2003, http://www.abanet.org/irr/hr/spring03/livingdonors.html (accessed January 28, 2008).

4. Vance Hartke, from U.S. Senate Finance Committee report, September 26, 1972, as quoted in *Biomedical Politics*, ed. Kathi E. Hanna (Washington, D.C.: National Academies Press, 1991), 192, http://books.nap.edu/openbook.php?record_id=1793&page=192 (accessed January 28, 2008). The term "artificial kidney" refers to dialysis.

5. Robert M. Ball, "Social Security Amendments of 1972: Summary and Legislative History," *In-Depth Research: Legislative History*, Social Security Online, http://www.ssa.gov/history/1972amend.html (accessed October 2, 2007); Hanna, ed., *Biomedical Politics*, 200.

6. U.S. Renal Data System, *Medicare Costs for ESRD*, http://www.usrds.org/2006/ref/K_econ_06.pdf (accessed February 7, 2008).

7. Kant Patel and Mark E. Rushefsky, *Health Care Policies in an Age of New Technologies* (Armonk, N.Y.: M. E. Sharpe, 2002), 74.

8. National Organ Transplant Act (NOTA), Pub. L. No. 98–507, sec. 301 (1984). Some commentators also point to the founding in 1983 of the International Kidney Exchange by Virginia physician H. Barry Jacobs as having spurred the enactment of NOTA; see Shapiro, "Legal Issues in Payment of Living Donors"; Jennifer L. Hurley, "Cashing In on the Transplant List: An Argument against Offering Valuable Compensation for the Donation of Organs," *Journal of High Technology Law* 4, no. 1 (2004): 126n61; and Gwen Mayes, "Buying and Selling Organs for Transplantation in the United States," *Medscape Transplantation* 4, no. 2 (December 9, 2003). Jacobs's business (which ultimately failed) acted as a broker between kidney patients who wished to buy organs from live donors, and individuals—many of them poor third-world residents—who wished to sell their kidneys. While the enterprise did lead to considerable debate about the ethics of offering financial incentives for donor organs, congressional hearings on arranging a nationwide system for organ distribution had already been held before the International Kidney Exchange came to light. Its emergence did, however, bring national attention to the debate on buying and selling organs, and, according to Mayes, it prompted the inclusion in NOTA of a ban on organ purchases. See Mayes, "Buying and Selling Organs for Transplantation," as well as chapter 8 and the conclusion.

9. U.S. House of Representatives, Committee on Energy and Commerce, Subcommittee on Health and the Environment, *National Organ Transplant Act: Hearing Before the Subcommittee on Health and the Environment of the House Committee on Energy and Commerce*, 98th Cong., 1st sess. (1983), transcript of July 23, 1983 radio broadcast by President Ronald Reagan, 4–5.

10. U.S. House of Representatives, Committee on Science and Technology, Subcommittee on Investigations and Oversight, *Organ Transplants: Hearing before the Subcommittee on Investigations and Oversight of the House Committee on Science and Technology*, 98th Cong., 1st sess. (1983), statement of Donald Denny, director of organ procurement, Transplant Foundation, University of Pittsburgh.

11. U.S. House of Representatives, Committee on Energy and Commerce, Subcommittee on Health and the Environment, *National Organ Transplant Act: Hearing Before the Subcommittee on Health and the Environment of the House Committee on Energy and Commerce*, 98th Congress, 2d sess., February 9, 1984.

12. Jerold R. Mande (associate director for policy, Yale Cancer Center), email communication to the author, February 19, 2007. Recently, Mande pointed out that the subcommittee's concerns about the effect of payment on altruistic giving were focused on organs from the newly deceased, and that its findings might not bear on the question of whether compensated living donors would "crowd out" altruistic ones. "Living organ donation is different," Mande said. "Our investigation found that financial incentives were unlikely to be effective in increasing the cadaveric donor organ supply. At the time, living organ donation was generally limited to related individuals. A stronger case could

be made that markets or financial incentives could increase unrelated living donation." Mande, personal communication with Sally Satel, May 27, 2008. Furthermore, in the early 1980s when Mande and colleagues solicited reactions from transplant professionals, there was no nationally coordinated organ procurement and distribution system in place. Accordingly, transplant professionals anticipated that creating one would improve organ procurement and distribution markedly and, thus, had little sense of urgency regarding the need to explore novel procurement efforts (such as incentives). For more on the controversy surrounding the question of altruistic crowding out, see chapters 5, 6, and 7.

13. National Organ Transplant Act (NOTA), Pub. L. No. 98–507, sec. 301 (1984) sec. 274e.

14. Ibid.

15. U.S. Congressional Research Service, *CRS Report for Congress: Living Organ Donation and Valuable Consideration*, by Erin D. Williams, Bernice Reyes-Akinbileje, and Kathleen S. Swendiman, order code RL33902, March 8, 2007, 9, http://assets.opencrs.com/rpts/RL33902_20070308.pdf (accessed January 28, 2008).

16. Ibid., 10.

17. U.S. House of Representatives, Committee on Science and Technology, Subcommittee on Investigations, *Procurement and Allocation of Human Organs for Transplantation: Hearing Before the Subcommittee on Investigations and Oversight of the House Committee on Science and Technology*, 98th Congress, 1st sess., November 9, 1983, statements of Peter Dobrovitz, kidney recipient, Rochester, N.Y., 253; Marvin Brams, MD, College of Urban Affairs and Public Policy, University of Delaware, 256–58, 300–301; and H. Barry Jacobs, MD, medical director, International Kidney Exchange, Ltd., 258–68, 283–301. U.S. House of Representatives, Committee on Energy and Commerce, Subcommittee on Health and the Environment, *National Organ Transplant Act: Hearing Before the Subcommittee on Health and the Environment of the House Committee on Energy and Commerce*, 98th Cong., 2d sess., February 9, 1984, statement of H. Barry Jacobs, MD, medical director, International Kidney Exchange, Ltd., 238–50.

18. *Congressional Record*, daily ed., June 20 and 21, 1984.

19. National Organ Transplant Act, sec. 273 (b) (3) B and E.

20. Kathleen S. Andersen and Daniel M. Fox, "The Impact of Routine Inquiry Laws on Organ Donation," *Health Affairs* 7, no. 5 (Winter 1988): 65, http://content.healthaffairs.org/cgi/reprint/7/5/65.pdf (accessed October 15, 2007).

21. Omnibus Reconciliation Act of 1986, 42 U.S.C. sec. 1320b-8(a)(1)(A).

22. Omnibus Reconciliation Act of 1986, 42 U.S.C. sec. 1320b-8(a)(1)(B).

23. Uniform Law Commission, National Conference of Commissioners on Uniform State Laws, "New Revision to the Rules."

24. National Conference of Commissioners on Uniform State Laws, Uniform Anatomical Gift Act (1987), approved and recommended for enactment by all the states at NCCUSL's ninety-sixth annual conference, Newport Beach, Calif., July 31–August 7,

1987, http://www.law.upenn.edu/bll/archives/ulc/fnact99/uaga87.htm (accessed October 15, 2007).

25. *Encyclopedia of Everyday Law*, s.v. "Organ Donation," eNotes.com, 2006, http://law.enotes.com/everyday-law-encyclopedia/organ-donation (accessed January 28, 2008).

26. National Conference of Commissioners on Uniform State Laws, Uniform Anatomical Gift Act of 1987.

27. Uniform Law Commissioners, National Conference of Commissioners on Uniform State Laws, "New Revision to the Rules."

28. *Encyclopedia of Everyday Law*, s.v. "Organ Donation."

29. Ibid.

30. Federal Patient Self Determination Act of 1991, 42 U.S.C. sec. 1395cc, 42 U.S.C. 1396a.

31. *Encyclopedia of Everyday Law*, s.v. "Organ Donation."

32. Organ Donor Leave Act, Pub. L. No. 106-56 (1999).

33. U.S. Congressional Research Service, *Living Organ Donation and Valuable Consideration*, 3.

34. Eventually a new version was proposed as H.R. 3926.

35. Organ Donation and Recovery Improvement Act, S. 573, 108th Cong., 1st sess. (March 6, 2003).

36. Organ Donation and Recovery Improvement Act, Pub. L. No. 108-216 (2004).

37. F. Delmonico, letter to the editor, *Kidney International* 70 (2006): 605–6, http://www.nature.com/ki/journal/v70/n3/full/5001689a.html (accessed January 28, 2008).

38. National Living Donor Assistance Center, program background, http://www.livingdonorassistance.org/theprogram/background.aspx (accessed June 12, 2008).

39. Uniform Law Commissioners, National Conference of Commissioners on Uniform State Laws, "New Revision to the Rules."

40. Uniform Law Commissioners, National Conference of Commissioners on Uniform State Laws, "ABA Approves Four Uniform Acts: New Act on Organ Donation among Acts Approved," press release, February 12, 2007, http://www.nccusl.org/Update/DesktopModules/NewsDisplay.aspx?ItemID=178 (accessed October 3, 2007).

41. See http://www.nccusl.org/Update/uniformact_factsheets/uniformacts-fs-uaga.asp (accessed November 3, 2008).

42. U.S. Congressional Research Service, *Living Organ Donation and Valuable Consideration*, summary.

43. Charlie W. Norwood Living Organ Donation Act, Pub. L. No. 110-144 (2007).

44. Republican Study Committee, "H.R. 710—Living Kidney Organ Donation Act," *Legislative Bulletin*, March 6, 2007, 10, www.house.gov/hensarling/rsc/doc/LB_030607_suspensions.doc (accessed June 25, 2008).

45. President's Council on Bioethics, "Caring for Living Donors and Transplant Recipients: Five Policy Proposals," staff discussion paper by Sam Crowe and Erin

Cohen, http://www.bioethics.gov/background/caring_for_living_donors.html (accessed January 28, 2008).

46. Transplant Living, "Financial Aspects: State Tax Deductions and Donor Leave Laws," http://www.transplantliving.org/livingdonation/financialaspects/statetax.aspx (accessed January 28, 2008). The states are Arkansas, Georgia, Iowa, Minnesota, Mississippi, New Mexico, New York, North Dakota, Oklahoma, Utah, and Wisconsin.

47. National Conference of State Legislatures, "State Leave Laws Related to Medical Donors," http://www.ncsl.org/programs/employ/Leave-medicaldonors.htm (accessed February 14, 2008).

48. Transplant Living, "Financial Aspects." The states are Arkansas, Connecticut, Illinois, Louisiana, Maine, Minnesota, Nebraska, and Oregon.

49. U.S. House of Representatives, Committee on Energy and Commerce, Subcommittee on Oversight and Investigations, *Assessing Initiatives to Increase Organ Donations: Hearing Before the Subcommittee on Oversight and Investigations of the House Committee on Energy and Commerce*, 108th Cong., 1st sess., June 3, 2003, statement of Tim Olsen, community development coordinator, Wisconsin Donor Network, 48.

50. Kevin B. O'Reilly, "Prison Organ Donation Proposal Worrisome," *Amednews.com*, April 9, 2007, http://www.ama-assn.org/amednews/2007/04/09/prsb0409.htm (accessed February 1, 2008).

51. Georgia Department of Driver Services, Organ Donor Program, June 30, 2005, http://www.dds.ga.gov/drivers/DLdata.aspx?con=1747097292&ty=dl (accessed February 1, 2008).

52. See chapter 8.

53. Hastings Center, "Tax Incentives: A Market Solution to the Kidney Shortage?" *Hasting Center Report* 11, no. 5 (October 1981), 3.

54. The Legislative Resource Center of the United States House of Representatives Library, personal communication with Kristin Viswanathan, Sept. 17, 2008.

55. H.R. 3471, 106th Cong, 1st sess. (November 18, 1999).

56. H.R. 5224, 107th Cong., 2d sess. (July 25, 2002), H.R. 2856, 108th Cong., 1st sess. (July 24, 2003).

57. S. 2495, 103rd Cong., 2d sess. (October 3, 1994), H.R. 1012, 103rd Cong., 1st sess. (February 18, 1993), H.R. 2551, 104th Cong., 1st sess. (October 26, 1995), S. 1713, 104th Cong., 2d sess. (April 29, 1996), H.R. 1505, 105th Cong., 1st sess. (April 30, 1997), S. 636, 105th Cong., 1st sess. (April 23, 1997), H.R. 941, 106th Cong., 1st sess. (March 2, 1999), S. 499, 106th Cong., 1st sess. (March 2, 1999), H.R. 708, 107th Cong., 1st sess. (February 14, 2001), S. 325, 107th Cong., 1st sess. (February 14, 2001), H.R. 1251, 108th Cong., 1st sess. (March 12, 2003), S. 572, 108th Cong., 1st sess. (March 6, 2003), H.R. 4753, 109th Cong., 2d sess. (February 14, 2006), S. 2283, 109th Cong., 2d sess. (February 14, 2006), S. 1062, 110th Cong., 1st sess. (March 29, 2007), H.R. 1764, 110th Cong., 1st sess. (March 29, 2007).

58. H.R. 1857, 106th Cong., 1st sess. (May 18, 1999).

59. The credit would presumably go to the deceased individual's beneficiaries or estate.

60. H.R. 4048, 106th Cong., 2d sess. (March 21, 2000); H.R. 1872, 107th Cong., 1st sess. (May 16, 2001).

61. H.R. 5436, 106th Cong., 2d sess. (October 10, 2000); H.R. 2090, 107th Cong., 1st sess. (June 6, 2001).

62. H.R. 2474, 109th Cong., 1st sess. (May 19, 2005), H.R. 1035, 110th Cong., 1st sess. (February 13, 2007); U.S. Congressional Research Service, *CRS Report for Congress*, 5.

63. An exception is the failed Help Organ Procurement Expand Act; see above.

64. See previous discussion, and chapter 8.

65. U.S. House of Representatives, Committee on Commerce, Subcommittee on Health and Environment, *Putting Patients First: Increasing Organ Supply for Transplantation: Hearing Before the Subcommittee on Health and Environment, of the Committee on Commerce*, 106th Cong., 1st sess., April 15, 1999, 58.

66. Ibid.

67. Ibid., 65. LifeLink's strategies involved simplifying the donation process, improving the training of hospital employees who approach bereaved families for donor organs, and establishing a strong liaison program between hospitals and organ procurement organizations. Ibid., 14.

68. Ibid., 70–71.

69. Ibid., 67–68.

70. U.S. House of Representatives, Committee on Energy and Commerce, Subcommittee on Oversight and Investigations, *Assessing Initiatives*, 53–54.

71. Ibid., 22–23.

72. Ibid., 43.

73. Ibid., 62.

74. American Society of Transplant Surgeons, "American Society of Transplant Surgeons Statement on Solicitation of Donor Organs," http://findarticles.com/p/articles/mi_m0YUG/is_23_14/ai_n17208367 (accessed January 31, 2008).

75. U.S. House of Representatives, Committee on Energy and Commerce, Subcommittee on Oversight and Investigations, *Assessing Initiatives*, 62. The ASTS may have been a bit leery of having its position misinterpreted, as it had been a year previously. In 2002, the society's ethics panel had unanimously opposed the exchange of money for donor organs but said, as Shaked repeated at the 2003 hearing, that a small reimbursement for funeral expenses would be appropriate as a sign of gratitude to the donor's family. Members must have been dismayed when the *Medical Post* reported the panel's supposed support for financial compensation for families of deceased donors under the headline, "Paying for Organs." James F. Childress and Catharyn T. Liverman, eds., *Organ Donation: Opportunities for Action* (Washington, D.C.: National Academies Press, 2006), 249.

76. U.S. House of Representatives, Committee on Energy and Commerce, Subcommittee on Oversight and Investigations, *Assessing Initiatives*, 51–54.

77. Ibid.

78. Ibid., 67.

Appendix B

1. G. E. W. Wolstenholme and Maeve O'Conner (eds.), *Ethics in Medical Progress: With Special Reference to Transplantation* (London: J. & A. Churchill, Ltd., 1966), 35.

2. U.S. House of Representatives, Committee on Energy and Commerce, Subcommittee on Health and the Environment: *Hearings on the National Organ Transplant Act*, 98th Cong., 1st sess., July 1983, statement of Thomas E. Starzl, 225.

3. Jesse Dukeminier Jr., "Supplying Organs for Transplantation," *Michigan Law Review* 68, no. 5 (April 1970): 811; Simon Rottenberg, "The Production and Exchange of Body Parts," in *Towards Liberty: Essays on Honor of Ludwig von Mises on the Occasion of his 90th Birthday*, September 29, 1971, ed. Friedrich A. von Hayek (Menlo Park, Calif.: Institute for Humane Studies, 1971), 326; Timothy M. Hartman, "The Buying and Selling of Human Organs From the Living: Why Not?" *Akron Law Review* 13, no. 1 (1979): 152–74.

4. Marvin Brams, "Transplantable Human Organs: Should Their Sale Be Authorized by State Statutes?" *American Journal of Law and Medicine* 2, no. 3 (Summer 1977): 183–95. Economist Marvin Brams at the University of Delaware laid out a proposal for a "combined altruistic-market system" that would be designed and administered at the state level through statutory provisions.

5. The inexorable widening of the gap between supply and demand can be documented with depressing accuracy from 1987, the year in which the national registry of patients in need of organs was first published.

6. Harry Schwartz, "Providing Incentives for Organ Donations," *Wall Street Journal*, July 25, 1983, 10.

7. Council of the Transplantation Society, "Commercialisation in Transplantation: The Problems and Some Guidelines for Practice," *Lancet* 326, no. 8457 (September 1985): 715. The Transplantation Society no longer supports this view; see chapter 4.

8. Richard Schwindt and Aidan R. Vining, "Proposal for a Future Delivery Market for Transplant Organs," *Journal of Health Politics, Policy and Law* 11, no. 3 (Fall 1986): 483–500. See Henry Hansmann, "The Economics and Ethics of Markets for Human Organs," *Journal of Health Politics, Policy and Law* 14, no. 1 (Spring 1989): 57–85; Lloyd R. Cohen, "Increasing the Supply of Transplant Organs: The Virtues of a Futures Market," *George Washington Law Review* 58, no. 1 (November 1989): 1–51.

9. James F. Blumstein and Frank A. Sloan (eds.), *Organ Transplant Policy: Issues and Prospects* (Durham, N.C.: Duke University Press, 1989). In a chapter in this symposium volume entitled, "Ethical Criteria for Procuring and Distributing Organs for Transplantation" (87–113), James F. Childress states, "If a system of donation with various modifications proves to be insufficiently effective, then transfer by sales could be tried, even though it would not express the value of altruism that leads many to favor the gift relationship" (101). And, according to one reviewer, "The implicit message I get from [the Blumstein and Sloan] book is that it is time to move beyond such hand-wringing, but the system is probably already inextricably snared by the emerging appa-

ratchiks." See Aidan Vining, "Organ Transplantation Policy: Issues and Prospects," *Journal of Policy Analysis and Management* 10, no. 3 (Summer 1991): 505–6.

10. Thomas G. Peters, "Life or Death: The Issue of Payment in Cadaveric Organ Donation," *Journal of the American Medical Association* 265, no. 10 (March 1991): 1302.The next year, Canadian transplant surgeon Abdullah Daar published a paper entitled "Rewarded Gifting"; see *Transplantation Proceedings* 24, no. 5 (October 1992): 2207–11.

11. Yankelovich Clancy Shulman, "The Ethical Questions of Organ Donation," poll conducted for *Time*/CNN, June 4–5, 1991.

12. "Old Taboo Falls at NKF Consensus Conference Meeting; Experts Okay Financial Incentives for Donation," *Transplant News* 1, no. 14 (March 14, 1991). P.1 The panel recommended a poll be conducted prior to implementation of these projects. This was the joint UNOS/NKF survey cited in appendix C.

13. U.S. Department of Health and Human Services, Public Health Service, *Proceedings of the Surgeon General's Workshop on Increasing Organ Donation* (Washington, D.C., July 8–10, 1991), http://profiles.nlm.nih.gov/NN/B/C/Y/P/_/nnbcyp.pdf (accessed June 3, 2008).

14. P. M. Khanna, "Scarcity of Organs for Transplant Sparks a Move to Legalize Financial Incentives," *Wall Street Journal,* September 8, 1992, B1, B6. See also D. Joralemon, "Organ Wars: The Battle for Body Parts," *Medical Anthropology Quarterly* 9, no. 3 (1995): 335–56.

15. A. Bruce Bowden, quoted in Peter S. Young, "Moving to Compensate Families in Human-Organ Market," *New York Times*, July 8, 1994.

16. UNOS Ethics Committee, "Financial Incentives for Organ Donation: A Report of the UNOS Ethics Payment Subcommittee," June 30, 1993, http://home.columbus. rr.com/mhollowa/financial.txt (accessed October 15, 2007).

17. American Medical Association, Council on Ethical and Judicial Affairs, "Financial Incentives for Organ Procurement. Ethical Aspects of Future Contracts for Cadaveric Donors," *Archives of Internal Medicine* 155, no. 6 (March 1995): 581.

18. David J. Rothman, Eric Rose, Tsuyoshi Awaya, B. Cohen, Abdullah S. Daar, Sergey L. Dzemeshkevich, C. J. Lee, Robin Munro, Hernan Reyes, Sheila M. Rothman, K. F. Schoen, Nancy Scheper-Hughes, Ziva Shapira, and Heiner Smit, "The Bellagio Task Force Report on Transplantation, Bodily Integrity, and the International Traffic in Organs," *Transplantation Proceedings* 29, no. 6 (September 1997): 2741.

19. Sheryl Gay Stolberg, "Pennsylvania Set to Break Taboo on Rewards for Organ Donations," *New York Times*, May 6, 1999, A1.

20. Eli A. Friedman and Amy L. Friedman, "Payment for Donor Kidneys: Pros and Cons," *Kidney International* 69, no. 6 (March 2006): 960–2; Anthony P. Monaco, "Rewards for Organ Donation: The Time Has Come," *Kidney International* 69, no. 6 (March 2006): 955–57; Muthu Krishna Mani, "Payment for Donor Kidneys," *Kidney International* 70, no. 3 (August 2006): 603; Mario Abbud-Filho, H. H. Campos, Valter Duro Garcia, and J. O. Medina Pestana, "Payment for Donor Kidneys: Only Cons," *Kidney International* 70, no. 3

(August 2006): 603; Eli A. Friedman and Amy L. Friedman, "Response to 'Payment for Donor Kidneys: Only Cons,'" *Kidney International* 70, no. 3 (August 2006): 604; Charles J. Diskin and David L. Kaserman, "The Transplant Donor Payment Debate," *Kidney International* 70, no. 3 (August 2006): 604; Francis Delmonico, "The Transplant Donor Payment Debate," *Kidney International* 70, no. 3 (August 2006): 605; David J. Undis, "Response to 'Voluntary Reciprocal Altruism: A Novel Strategy to Encourage Decreased Organ Donation,'" *Kidney International* 70, no. 3 (August 2006): 606; Donald W. Landry, "Response to 'Voluntary Reciprocal Altruism: A Novel Strategy to Encourage Decreased Organ Donation,'" *Kidney International* 70, no. 3 (August 2006): 606; Hippen, "Preventive Measures May Not Reduce Demand"; Aaron Spital, "Conscription of Cadaveric Organs for Transplantation: Time to Start Talking About It," *Kidney International* 70, no. 3 (August 2006): 607; Alexandra K. Glazier and Francis L. Delmonico, "Response to 'Conscription of Cadaveric Organs for Transplantation: Time to Start Talking About It,'" *Kidney International* 70, no. 3 (August 2006): 607; Randy Cohen, "Organ Sales: Compromising Ethics," *Kidney International* 70, no. 3 (August 2006): 608; Meyer D. Lifschitz, "Paying for Kidneys for Transplantation," *Kidney International* 70, no. 3 (August 2006): 608; Benjamin E. Hippen and Robert S. Gaston, "The Conspicuous Costs of More of the Same," *American Journal of Transplantation* 6, no. 7 (July 2006): 1503–4; Richard J. Howard, "Missed Opportunities: The Institute of Medicine Report: Organ Donation: Opportunities for Action, *American Journal of Transplantation* 7, no. 1 (January 2007): 14–16; Abdallah S. Daar, "The Case for a Regulated System of Living Kidney Sales," *Nature Clinical Practice Nephrology* 2, no. 11 (November 2006): 600–601; James Stacey Taylor, "Black Markets, Transplant Kidneys and Interpersonal Coercion," *Journal of Medical Ethics* 32, no. 12 (December 2006): 698–701; "What's Wrong with Selling Kidneys?" *ScienceDaily,* June 15, 2008 http://www.sciencedaily.com/releases/ 2008/06/ 080613111854.htm; Kuldip P. Anand, Ajit Kashyap, and Surekha Kashyap, "Thinking the Unthinkable: Selling Kidneys," *British Medical Journal* 333, no. 7559 (July 2006): 149; Michael M. Friedlaender, "The Right to Sell or Buy a Kidney: Are We Failing Our Patients?" *Lancet* 359, no. 9310 (March 2002): 971–73; Mary Simmerling, Peter Angelos, John Franklin, and Michael Abecassis, "The Commercialization of Human Organs for Transplantation: The Current Status of the Ethical Debate," *Current Opinion in Organ Transplantation* 11, no. 2 (April 2006): 130–35; Arthur J. Matas, "The Case for Living Kidney Sales: Rationale, Objections and Concerns," *American Journal of Transplantation* 4, no. 12 (December 2004): 2007–2017; John Harris and Charles Erin, "An Ethically Defensible Market in Organs," *British Medical Journal* 325, no. 7368 (July 2002): 114–15.

21. Donald Joralemon, "Shifting Ethics: Debating the Incentive Question in Organ Transplantation," *Journal of Medical Ethics* 27, no. 1 (February 2001): 30.

22. J. Warren, "ACOT Recommends HHS Demonstration Project on Financial Incentives," *Transplant News* 12, no. 22 (November 27, 2002). P. 1 The ethics committee of the ASTS was in favor of a token reward to families who donate; this offer was explicitly meant as a "thank you," not an inducement. See J. Warren, "ASTA Ethic Committee Endorses Pilot Program to Test Financial Incentives to Increase Organ Donation," *Transplant News* 12, no. 10 (May 28, 2002): 1.

23. Deborah Josefson, "AMA Considers Whether to Pay for Donation of Organs," *British Medical Journal* 324, no. 7353 (June 2002): 1541.

24. *Transplant News*, "Resolutions Passed by Participants Attending International Congress on Ethics in Organ Transplantation, December 10–13, Munich, Germany," January 15, 2003.

25. U.S. House of Representatives, Committee on Energy and Commerce, Subcommittee on Oversight and Investigations, *Assessing Initiatives to Increase Organ Donations*, 108th Cong., 1st sess., June 3, 2003, http://energycommerce.house.gov/reparchives/108/Hearings/06032003hearing946/print.htm (accessed April 2, 2008). Robert M. Sade testified on behalf of the American Medical Association: "We have noted that financial incentives might be an important motivational factor in the context of cadaveric organ donation but that it remains inadequately explored because of federal prohibition. In our view, such incentives are not intrinsically unethical even though they are counter to current customs, and, if proven effective, could save the lives of many patients suffering from end-stage organ failure."

26. Ibid. Regarding UNOS, see 84; regarding AOPO, see 22–23.

27. *Transplant News* 14, no. 21 (November 16, 2004): 3.

28. Ibid.

29. Michele Goodwin, *Black Markets: The Supply and Demand of Body Parts* (New York: Cambridge University Press, 2006); Mark J. Cherry, *Kidney for Sale by Owner: Human Organs*, Transplantation, and the Market (Washington, D.C.: Georgetown University Press, 2005); James Stacey Taylor, *Stakes And Kidneys: Why Markets in Human Body Parts Are Morally Imperative* (Burlington, Vt.: Ashgate Publishing, 2005).

30. Richard N. Fine (president, American Society of Transplantation), presidential address, 2006 World Transplant Congress, July 19, 2006.

31. Anthony Monaco, "Financial Rewards for Organ Donation: Are We Getting Closer?" *Expert Review of Pharmacoeconomics & Outcomes Research* 7, no. 4 (August 2007): 303–7.

32. Arthur Matas (president, American Society of Transplant Surgeons), personal communication with the author, February 8, 2007.

33. American Medical Association. Financial incentives could improve organ donation and reduce donor-recipient gap, June 16, 2003 at http://www.ama-assn.org/ama/pub/category/18674.html, (accessed June 27, 2008).

34. Letter from AAKP, Roberta Wager, President, dated Sept. 22, 2008 (on file with author); letter from AST, Barbara Murphy, MD, President, dated Sept. 22, 2008 (on file with author).

Appendix C

1. Unless otherwise noted, all polls mentioned in this appendix are of representative random samples of American adults eighteen years of age or older.

2. Yankelovich Clancy Shulman, "The Ethical Questions of Organ Donation," poll conducted for *Time*/CNN, June 4–5, 1991.

3. Poll commissioned by the Health Care Financing Administration, as cited in Jeffrey M. Prottas, "Buying Human Organs: Evidence that Money Doesn't Change Everything," *Transplantation* 53, no. 6 (June 1992): 1371–73.

4. United Network for Organ Sharing, "Public Attitudes on Organ Donation: Quantitative Results of a UNOS/NKF Study," *UNOS Update*, 1992.

5. "Nearly Half of Americans Support Some Kind of Incentive for Donation," *Transplant News* 2, no. 23 (December 17, 1992): 2.

6. Beckey Bright, "Americans Are Divided on Offering Financial Incentives to Organ Donors," *Wall Street Journal Online*, May 17, 2007, http://online.wsj.com/article_print/SB117889765086700017.html (accessed March 3, 2008). The survey's design implied a traditional free market, which would be advantageous to the wealthy because they could afford to purchase organs. About 70 percent agreed that incentives would benefit the rich, and the poor would "resort to organ donation as a means to make money."

7. Alex Guttman and Ronald D. Guttman, "Attitudes of Healthcare Professionals and the Public towards the Sale of Kidneys for Transplantation," *Journal of Medical Ethics* 19, no. 3 (1993): 151.

8. A. Frank Adams III, A. H. Barnett, and David L. Kaserman, "Markets for Organs: The Question of Supply," *Contemporary Economic Policy* 17, no. 2 (April 1999): 147–55.

9. Cindy L. Bryce, Laura A. Siminoff, Peter A. Ubel, H. Nathan, Arthur L. Caplan, and Robert M. Arnold, "Do Incentives Matter? Providing Benefits to Families of Organ Donors," *American Journal of Transplantation* 5, no. 12 (December 2005): 2999–3007.

10. Ashwini R. Sehgal, S. O. LeBeau, and Stuart J. Youngner, "Dialysis Patient Attitudes toward Financial Incentives for Kidney Donation," *American Journal of Kidney Diseases* 29, no. 3 (March 1997): 410–18.

11. L. Ebony Boulware, Misty U. Troll, and Nae Y. Wang, "Public Attitudes toward Incentives for Organ Donation: A National Study of Different Racial/Ethnic and Income Groups," *American Journal of Transplantation* 6, no. 11 (November 2006): 2774–85. Note that despite the title of the article, which incorporates the word "incentives," study subjects were merely queried as to whether there should be rewards for acts of donation already committed, not whether an offer of material gain would enhance willingness of oneself or others to give.

12. Boulware et al. did not provide the actual percentages of African Americans (total n=102) and Hispanics (total n =130) in the study who said they were willing to be living donors.

13. The poll was commissioned by the Erasmus Medical Center. Leonieke Kranenburg, Andre Schram, Willij Zuidema, Wilem Weimar, et al., "Public Survey of Financial Incentives for Kidney Donation," *Nephrology Dialysis Transplantation* 23, no. 3 (2008): 1039–42. Most respondents believed that benefits would not influence their own behavior, but among those who said that they would make a difference, the net effect was to encourage donation; see Bryce et al., "Do Incentives Matter?"

14. William DeJong, Jessica Drachman, Steven L. Gortmaker, Carol Beasley, and Michael J. Evanisko, "Options for Increasing Organ Donation: The Potential Role of

Incentives, Standardized Hospital Procedures, and Public Education to Promote Family Discussion," *Milbank Quarterly* 73, no. 3 (1995): 463–79.

15. Partnership for Organ Donation and the Harvard School of Public Health, "The American Public's Attitudes toward Organ Donation and Transplantation," 1993, table 32, http://www.transweb.org/reference/articles/gallup_survey/gallup_index.html (accessed March 3, 2008).

16. U.S. Department of Health and Human Services, Health Resources and Services Administration, Division of Transplantation, *2005 National Survey of Organ and Tissue Donation Attitudes and Behaviors*, conducted by the Gallup Organization, Summer/Fall 2005, 24, http://www.organdonor.gov/survey2005 (accessed July 7, 2008).

17. John D. Jasper, Carol A. Nickerson, John C. Hershey, and David A. Asch, "The Public's Attitudes toward Incentives for Organ Donation," *Transplantation Proceedings* 31, no. 5 (August 1999): 2181–84.

18. Bryce et al., "Do Incentives Matter?"

19. James R. Rodrigue, Danielle L. Cornell, and Richard J. Howard, "Attitudes toward Financial Incentives, Donor Authorization, and Presumed Consent among Next-of-Kin Who Consented vs. Refused Organ Donation," *Transplantation* 91, no. 9 (May 2006): 1249–56.

20. Gill Haddow, "Because You're Worth It? The Taking and Selling of Transplantable Organs," *Journal of Medical Ethics* 32, no. 6 (2006): 324–28.

21. See note 6, above.

Appendix D

1. United Network for Organ Sharing, "Summary Statements of Various Religious Groups About Organ and Tissue Donation," October 24, 2001, http://www.unos.org/news/newsDetail.asp?id=236 (accessed April 7, 2008); Canadian Medical Association, "Religious Leaders Give Organ Donation a Boost," *Canadian Medical Association Journal* 157, no. 10 (November 1997): 1338.

2. Susan L. Mayer, "Thoughts on the Jewish Perspective Regarding Organ Transplantation," *Journal of Transplant Coordination* 7, no. 2 (June 1997): 67–71; Z. H. Rappaport and Isabelle T. Rappaport, "Principles and Concepts of Brain Death and Organ Donation: The Jewish Perspective," *Child's Nervous System* 14, no. 8 (August, 1998): 381–83; Rav Moshe David Tendler, "Halachic Death Means Brain Death," *Jewish Review*, January–February 1990, 6, 20. According to these articles, there is some controversy among Jews over the (mistaken) belief that Jewish law forbids cadaveric organ donation because of rules against the desecration of the body after death, and that Jewish law only recognizes cardiac death (cessation of heartbeat), rather than brain stem failure, as death. Another misconception is that Jewish law prohibits autopsy, but this proscription is waived if it is required by law to solve a crime.

3. Patrick Henry Reardon, "The Commerce of Human Body Parts: An Eastern Orthodox Response," *Christian Bioethics* 6, no. 2 (August 2000): 205–13; Nicholas

Capaldi, "A Catholic Perspective on Organ Sales," *Christian Bioethics* 6, no. 2 (August 2000): 139–51; James F. Childress, "Protestant Perspective on Organ Donation," in *Pediatric Brain Death and Organ/Tissue Retrieval: Medical, Ethical, and Legal Aspects*, ed. Howard H. Kaufman (New York: Plenum Publishing Corporation, 1989), 48.

4. Shlomo H. Goren, *Torat Harefuah* (Jerusalem, 2000), as quoted in Richard V. Grazi and Joel B. Wolowelsky, "Nonaltruistic Kidney Donations in Contemporary Jewish Law and Ethics," *Transplantation* 75, no. 2 (January 2003): 251

5. Abraham S. Abraham, "Nishmat Avraham IV," *Hoshen Mishpat* 420, no. 3, as quoted in Grazi and Wolowelsky, "Nonaltruistic Kidney Donations in Contemporary Jewish Law."

6. Yisrael Meir Lau, "Selling Organs for Transplantation," *Tehumin* 18 (1998): 125, as quoted in Grazi and Wolowelsky, "Nonaltruistic Kidney Donations in Contemporary Jewish Law," 252; note also that Lau stated that the ruling is based on a discussion by the late rabbinical arbiters rabbis Shlomo Zalman Auerbach and Shaul Yisraeli. Judy Siegel, "Chief Rabbi OKs Sale of Human Organs," *Jerusalem Post*, January 8, 1998. According to Daniel Eisenberg, an American physician and expert in Jewish medical ethics, "If allowing payments for organs with proper safeguards would increase the number of lives saved, then Jewish law would sanction such an approach." See Daniel Eisenberg, "Live Organ Donation: Does Jewish Law Permit Donating an Organ? What About Selling One?" *Aish HaTorah* Online, http://www.aish.com/societyWork/science-nature/Live_Organ_Donation.asp (accessed July 3, 2008).

7. J. D. Kunin, "The Search for Organs: Halachic Perspectives on Altruistic Giving and the Selling of Organs," *Journal of Medical Ethics*, 31 (2005): 269–72.

8. Jayson Rapoport, Alexander Kagan, and Michael M. Friedlaender, "Legalizing the Sale of Kidneys for Transplantation: Suggested Guidelines," *Israel Medical Association Journal* 4, no. 12 (December 2002): 1132–34.

9. Daniel B. Sinclair, *Jewish Biomedical Law: Legal and Extra-Legal Dimensions* (New York: Oxford University Press, 2003), 243; Richard V. Grazi and Joel B. Wolowelsky, "Jewish Medical Ethics: Monetary Compensation for Donating Kidneys," *Israel Medical Association Journal* 6, no. 3 (March 2004): 185–88. The authors argue that Jewish ethics allow a lifesaving organ sale, provided there is no exploitation, informed consent is secured, and participants are compensated for pain and suffering.

10. Dariusch Atighetchi, "The Development of Organ Transplants," in *Islamic Bioethics: Problems and Perspectives*, 161–97 (New York: Springer, 2006).

11. Mohammad Mehdi Golmakani, Mohammad Hussein Niknam, and Kamyar M. Hedayat, "Transplantation Ethics from the Islamic Point of View," *Medical Science Monitor* 11, no. 4 (2005), RA105–9.

12. M. Al-Mousawi et al., "Views of Muslim Scholars on Organ Donation and Brain Death," *Transplantation Proceedings* 29, no. 8 (1997): 3217.

13. Atighetchi, "Development of Organ Transplants."

14. Muhammad Y. A. Abul-Fotouh, "Sale of Human Organs in the Balance of Legitimacy," presented at Medical Jurisprudence Third Symposium on "The Islamic

Vision of Some Medical Practices," April 18–21, 1987, http://www.islamselect.com/en/mat/63778 (accessed July 7, 2008).

15. Ibid.

16. Mokhtar al-Mahdi, "Donation, Sale, and Unbequeathed Possession of Human Organs," in *The Islamic Vision of Some Medical Practices*, ed. K. al-Mazkur, A. al-Saif, Ahmad Rajaii al-Gindi, and A. Abu-Ghudda (Kuwait: IOMS Publications, 1989), as quoted in Sahin Aksoy, "A Critical Approach to the Current Understanding of Islamic Scholars on Using Cadaver Organs Without Prior Permission," *Bioethics* 15, no. 5–6 (October 2001), 468–69.

17. Muhammad Sayed Tantawi, "Judgement on Sale or Donation of Human Organs," in *The Islamic Vision of Some Medical Practices*, ed. K. al-Mazkur et al., as quoted in Aksoy, "A Critical Approach," 469.

18. Atighetchi, "Development of Organ Transplants."

19. Diane M. Tober, "Kidneys and Controversies in the Islamic Republic of Iran: The Case of Organ Sale," *Body & Society* 13, no. 151 (2007): 151–71.

20. Benjamin E. Hippen, "Organ Sales and Moral Travails: Lessons from the Living Kidney Vendor Program in Iran," Cato Policy Analysis No. 614, Cato Institute, March 2008, http://www.cato.org/pubs/pas/html/pa-614/pa-614index.html (accessed April 7, 2008).

21. Ibid., 153.

22. Tober, "Kidneys and Controversies"; Alireza Bagheri, "Compensated Kidney Donation: An Ethical Review of the Iranian Model," *Kennedy Institute of Ethics Journal* 16, no. 3 (September 2006): 269–82.

23. Pius XII, address to the delegates of the Italian Association for Cornea Donors and the Italian Union for the Blind, May 14, 1956, *Acta Apostolicae Sedis* 48 (1956): 465, http://www.ewtn.com/library/curia/pcpaheal.htm (accessed July 7, 2008).

24. John Paul II, "Address of the Holy Father John Paul II to the 18th International Congress of the Transplantation Society," Rome, August 29, 2000, http://www.vatican.va/holy_father/john_paul_ii/speeches/2000/jul-sep/documents/hf_jp-ii_spe_20000829_transplants_en.html (accessed July 3, 2008). The pope is quoting his 1991 address "To Participants of the First International Congress of the Society for Organ Sharing," June 20, 1991, http://www.vatican.va/holy_father/john_paul_ii/speeches/1991/june/documents/hf_jp-ii_spe_19910620_trapianti_en.html (accessed July 7, 2008).

25. Ibid.

26. United States Conference of Catholic Bishops, "Ethical and Religious Directives for Catholic Health Care Services," 4th ed., Washington D.C., Directive 30 (June 15, 2001), http://www.usccb.org/bishops/directives.shtml#partthree (accessed July 14, 2008).

27. National Catholic Bioethics Center, statement on the "Regulated Market of Organ Sales," Philadelphia, March 15, 2006, http://www.ncbcenter.org/06-03-15%20-%20Organ%20Sale.asp (accessed July 14, 2008).

28. Michael Novak (George Frederick Jewett Scholar in Religion, Philosophy, and Public Policy, American Enterprise Institute), personal communication with the author, March 25, 2008.

29. Capaldi, "A Catholic Perspective on Organ Sales," 139, 145; see also Peter A. Clark, "Financial Incentives for Cadaveric Organ Donation: An Ethical Analysis," *Internet Journal of Law, Healthcare and Ethics* 4, no. 1 (2006): 1–20. Clark is a Jesuit priest who has conducted a secular analysis of the problem of deceased donation and concluded that "there is no reason why such incentives should not be initiated" (16).

30. Mark J. Cherry, *Kidney for Sale by Owner: Human Organs, Transplantation, and the Market* (Washington, D.C.: Georgetown University Press, 2005), 124.

31. Ibid., 137.

32. Joseph Boyle, "Personal Responsibility and Freedom in Health Matters: A Contemporary Natural Law Perspective," in *Persons and their Bodies: Rights, Responsibilities, and Relationships*, ed. Mark J. Cherry (Dordrecht, Netherlands: Kluwer Academic Press, 1999), 111–41, 136.

Index

About the Authors

David C. Cronin II is director of liver transplantation and an associate professor of surgery at the Medical College of Wisconsin.

Julio J. Elías is an assistant professor in the Economics Department at the University at Buffalo (State University of New York). He is also an affiliated researcher in the university's Center of Excellence on Human Capital and Economic Growth and Development. His recent work, with Gary S. Becker of the University of Chicago, has focused on markets for organs. He received his doctorate in economics from the University of Chicago in 2005.

Richard A. Epstein is James Parker Hall Distinguished Service Professor of Law at the University of Chicago and the Peter and Kirsten Senior Fellow at the Hoover Institution. He is the author of many books, including *Takings: Private Property and the Power of Eminent Domain* (1985) and *Mortal Peril: Our Inalienable Right to Health Care?* (1997).

Michele Goodwin holds joint professorships at the University of Minnesota Medical School and the School of Public Health. She is the author of *Black Markets: The Supply and Demand of Body Parts* (2006), *Baby Markets* (2009), and numerous other publications. Professor Goodwin's research spans the domains of law, biotechnology, science, and medicine.

Benjamin E. Hippen is a nephrologist specializing in kidney transplantation at the Carolinas Medical Center in Charlotte, North Carolina. Dr. Hippen is an associate editor for the *American Journal of Transplantation* and serves on the editorial board of the *Journal of Medicine and Philosophy*.

Elbert S. Huang is an assistant professor of medicine, research associate of the Center on Demography and Economics of Aging, and co-investigator of the Diabetes Research and Training Center at the University of Chicago. Dr. Huang is the lead University of Chicago investigator for the

NORC-University of Chicago Health Economics Team for the JDRF Artificial Pancreas Project.

Arthur J. Matas is a professor of surgery at the University of Minnesota Medical School and director of its Renal Transplant Program.

David O. Meltzer is an associate professor in the Department of Medicine and the Department of Economics and in the Graduate School of Public Policy Studies at the University of Chicago.

Sally Satel is a resident scholar at the American Enterprise Institute and a lecturer at the Yale University School of Medicine, Department of Psychiatry. Her interest in transplant policy stems from her experience as a recipient of a kidney in 2006.

Mary C. Simmerling is the assistant dean for research integrity and an assistant professor of public health at Weill Cornell Medical College, Cornell University. She received her doctorate in philosophy from the University of Illinois and completed a fellowship in clinical medical ethics in the University of Chicago's MacLean Center for Clinical Medical Ethics.

James Stacey Taylor is an assistant professor of philosophy at the College of New Jersey. He is the author of *Stakes and Kidneys: Why Markets in Human Body Parts Are Morally Imperative* (2005) and the editor of *Personal Autonomy: New Essays on Personal Autonomy and Its Roles in Contemporary Moral Philosophy* (2005).

Nidhi Thakur is a health economist with primary interests in the economics of health-related behavior. Her doctorate in economics is from the University of Arizona, and she was awarded a postdoctoral fellowship by the University of Chicago. She has taught economics in institutions of higher learning, including Barnard College at Columbia University.

Chad A. Thompson is a student at the New York University School of Law. He earned a BS from Vanderbilt University and an MA in applied economics from Johns Hopkins University.

Research Staff

Gerard Alexander
Visiting Scholar

Ali Alfoneh
Visiting Research Fellow

Joseph Antos
Wilson H. Taylor Scholar in Health
Care and Retirement Policy

Leon Aron
Resident Scholar

Michael Auslin
Resident Scholar

Jeffrey Azarva
Research Fellow

Claude Barfield
Resident Scholar

Michael Barone
Resident Fellow

Roger Bate
Resident Fellow

Walter Berns
Resident Scholar

Douglas J. Besharov
Joseph J. and Violet Jacobs
Scholar in Social Welfare Studies

Andrew G. Biggs
Resident Scholar

Edward Blum
Visiting Fellow

Dan Blumenthal
Resident Fellow

John R. Bolton
Senior Fellow

Karlyn Bowman
Senior Fellow

Alex Brill
Research Fellow

Richard Burkhauser
Visiting Scholar

John E. Calfee
Resident Scholar

Charles W. Calomiris
Visiting Scholar

Lynne V. Cheney
Senior Fellow

Steven J. Davis
Visiting Scholar

Mauro De Lorenzo
Resident Fellow

Christopher DeMuth
D. C. Searle Senior Fellow

Thomas Donnelly
Resident Fellow

Nicholas Eberstadt
Henry Wendt Scholar in Political
Economy

Mark Falcoff
Resident Scholar Emeritus

John C. Fortier
Research Fellow

Ted Frank
Resident Fellow; Director, AEI Legal
Center for the Public Interest

David Frum
Resident Fellow

David Gelernter
National Fellow

Reuel Marc Gerecht
Resident Fellow

Newt Gingrich
Senior Fellow

Robert A. Goldwin
Resident Scholar Emeritus

Scott Gottlieb, M.D.
Resident Fellow

Kenneth P. Green
Resident Scholar

Michael S. Greve
John G. Searle Scholar

Robert W. Hahn
Senior Fellow; Executive Director,
AEI Center for Regulatory and
Market Studies

Kevin A. Hassett
Senior Fellow; Director,
Economic Policy Studies

Steven F. Hayward
F. K. Weyerhaeuser Fellow

Robert B. Helms
Resident Scholar

Frederick M. Hess
Resident Scholar; Director,
Education Policy Studies

Ayaan Hirsi Ali
Resident Fellow

R. Glenn Hubbard
Visiting Scholar

Frederick W. Kagan
Resident Scholar

Leon R. Kass, M.D.
Hertog Fellow

Herbert G. Klein
National Fellow

Marvin H. Kosters
Resident Scholar Emeritus

Irving Kristol
Senior Fellow Emeritus

Desmond Lachman
Resident Fellow

Lee Lane
Resident Fellow

Adam Lerrick
Visiting Scholar

Philip I. Levy
Resident Scholar

James R. Lilley
Senior Fellow

Lawrence B. Lindsey
Visiting Scholar

John H. Makin
Visiting Scholar

N. Gregory Mankiw
Visiting Scholar

Aparna Mathur
Research Fellow

Lawrence M. Mead
Visiting Scholar

Allan H. Meltzer
Visiting Scholar

Thomas P. Miller
Resident Fellow

Hassan Mneimneh
Visiting Fellow

Charles Murray
W. H. Brady Scholar

Roger F. Noriega
Visiting Fellow

Michael Novak
George Frederick Jewett Scholar
in Religion, Philosophy, and
Public Policy

Norman J. Ornstein
Resident Scholar

Richard Perle
Resident Fellow

Tomas J. Philipson
Visiting Scholar

Alex J. Pollock
Resident Fellow

Vincent R. Reinhart
Resident Scholar

Michael Rubin
Resident Scholar

Sally Satel, M.D.
Resident Scholar

Gary J. Schmitt
Resident Scholar; Director,
Program on Advanced
Strategic Studies

David Schoenbrod
Visiting Scholar

Nick Schulz
DeWitt Wallace Fellow; Editor-in-Chief,
The American magazine

Joel M. Schwartz
Visiting Fellow

Kent Smetters
Visiting Scholar

Christina Hoff Sommers
Resident Scholar; Director,
W. H. Brady Program

Samuel Thernstrom
Resident Fellow; Director, AEI Press

Bill Thomas
Visiting Fellow

Richard Vedder
Visiting Scholar

Alan D. Viard
Resident Scholar

Peter J. Wallison
Arthur F. Burns Fellow in
Financial Policy Studies

David A. Weisbach
Visiting Scholar

Paul Wolfowitz
Visiting Scholar

John Yoo
Visiting Scholar

When Altruism Isn't Enough